Has Your Child Been Traumatized?

Has Your Child Been Traumatized?

How to Know and What to Do to Promote Healing and Recovery

Melissa Goldberg Mintz

Foreword by Jon G. Allen

THE GUILFORD PRESS
New York   London

Last digit is print number: 9   8   7   6   5   4   3   2   1

Library of Congress Cataloging-in-Publication Data is available from
the publisher.

ISBN 978-1-4625-4749-4 (paperback) — ISBN 978-1-4625-5051-7 (hardcover)

Contents

PART III
Responding to Behavioral Changes

PART IV
Parenting Plus

Author's Note

In this book, I alternate among masculine, feminine, and plural pronouns when referring to a single individual. The intention behind this word choice is to represent as many readers as possible as our language continues to evolve. I sincerely hope that all will feel included.

I use the terms *parent–child relationship* and *caregiver–child relationship* interchangeably in this book. These terms are meant to include any custodial guardians, such as foster parents, grandparents, or any adult primary caregiver with whom the child currently lives.

All illustrations of families in this book are composites of individuals whose personal information, including demographic details, has been altered to protect their identities.

Foreword

If you were drawn in by the title of this book, you have come to the right place. First, take a moment to appreciate yourself: if you are parenting a traumatized child, to some degree you share your child's plight—feeling challenged, stressed, and sometimes downright confused. Examining this book, you are searching for guidance, motivated by caring and a desire to understand and help your child. Like your child, you need to feel understood, and you will find that understanding here. You will resonate with other parents' experience that comes through the pages of this book. You will read that avoidance of painful feelings is a natural human response, but avoidance keeps us stuck. We must cope, and you are coping by seeking understanding here. Your child is fortunate to have your care.

You have come to the right author, Melissa Goldberg Mintz. Before I met her, I had been conducting educational groups for hospitalized patients on trauma and attachment relationships for more than two decades. Dr. Goldberg Mintz volunteered to colead one of these groups during her postdoctoral fellowship and, as you will see immediately in this book, she was a natural—engaging, compassionate, and knowledgeable. She observed and listened. She was eager to learn and to share her knowledge. She spoke plainly, not caught up in jargon or technical language. I felt privileged to conduct these educational groups; the patients graciously had been educating me for many years. To the benefit of her readers, Dr. Goldberg Mintz has made the most of this privilege, continuing to learn and teach. She is a true psychologist, integrating science and practice. Most important, her work and writing are infused with her humanity.

Many years ago, at the end of a talk I gave to patients' family members, a father in the back of the room stood up and exclaimed, "Doctor, isn't all you've said just common sense?" I replied, "You've understood me perfectly!" But I added that I consider common sense to be a high aspiration. You will find a lot of common sense in this book. Here is the gist that no amount of detail should obscure: Your relationship with your child makes the most important contribution to your child's healing and recovery. What we call "secure attachment" is the model. Securely attached children are confident that, when they feel threatened and distressed, their parent will be available and sensitively responsive to their feelings and struggles. Abundant research shows that children who count on the safe haven of secure attachment also feel confident in exploring the world, knowing that they can count on comfort and help when they need it. Being able to depend on your caring and understanding enables your child to be increasingly independent.

Here is more common sense that you will find in this book: The more you are able to cultivate your child's feeling of security with you in everyday interactions, the more your child will rely on you for comfort and help with their traumatic experience. Trust and security develop moment by moment from thousands upon thousands of interactions, beginning in the earliest days of infancy. But you might be looking at this book because you are having difficulty relating to your child's traumatic responses. For example, if your traumatized child is experiencing overwhelming emotions and engaging in alarming behavior, you will be challenged to respond mindfully and sensitively, despite your best intentions. Perfection is not an option—far from it. At times, you might feel frustrated, discouraged, and worn out. Muddling through will count as a success.

Reading this book, you will see that you are not alone, and you can benefit from Dr. Goldberg Mintz's experience and abundant examples of parents' struggles and successes. Attachment research yields hopeful results: We all become more securely attached when we feel emotionally connected with those we depend on. Sometimes, we and those who provide care must work at connecting, especially when trauma interferes. Sometimes we need expert help, and such help with fostering security has been shown to be effective. Insecurity can be transformed into security.

Common sense is necessary but not sufficient when you are raising a traumatized child. After many years of training and clinical practice, I joined a group of colleagues in developing a specialized inpatient treatment program for traumatized patients. We all learned that specialized expertise was essential, and I spent many additional years acquiring it by conducting psychotherapy, educating patients, doing research, and writing articles and books. As Dr. Goldberg Mintz also has done, I learned most from those who were most expert: patients who were suffering from trauma and finding ways of healing. If well-educated professionals have much to learn, so will those who are on the front lines in helping their traumatized children heal. You will need no background in psychology or mental health to understand this book. Dr. Goldberg Mintz conveys the essential knowledge clearly, relying on her extensive experience in educating patients and their family members.

Traumatic stress takes many forms and comes in varying degrees. Some children recover and heal more readily than others. Dr. Goldberg Mintz offers straightforward guidance about how much specialized help you and your child might need. Exposure to potentially traumatic events is ubiquitous, but most individuals do not become seriously ill; they recover with ordinary caring and the restoration of safety. Even under these typical circumstances, however, you will find it helpful to understand the usual patterns of response to these extremely stressful experiences and the best ways of providing needed understanding and care.

While recovery with usual care is the rule, parents also need to be aware of the potentially enduring disturbance and disruptive behaviors that can ensue from traumatic experiences. Dr. Goldberg

Mintz gives particular attention to these more problematic patterns of disturbance and the specialized treatment approaches that can bolster recovery. All specialized treatments require facing the traumatic feelings and memories as well as coming to some understanding of the events and their impact. Most important, all these treatment approaches require thinking and talking about these experiences and feelings with a caring and empathic person who understands trauma.

If your child needs specialized treatment, you will learn from this book that there are many different treatments on offer, and you will need guidance in finding a good fit, an approach that makes sense to you and your child. But you should be aware of the finding of many decades of careful research on psychotherapy: The *quality of the patient–therapist relationship* contributes more to the effectiveness of the psychotherapy than the particular methods and techniques the therapist employs. Moreover, to a large degree, the qualities of the therapeutic relationship are similar to the qualities of the parent–child relationship described so insightfully in this book. Furthermore, as a parent, you will be your child's primary resource in recovering from trauma—before, during, and after specialized treatment. This book provides expert guidance for your role in healing and also provides information about how to access professional help.

With its extensive focus on infancy and early childhood, attachment research has been conducted largely with mothers. You should know that additional research shows the same pattern of findings for fathers and other primary caregivers. In an educational group for patients, with parents in the room in mind, I raised the question "What do parents need in order to foster secure attachment in the child?" The answer was obvious: secure attachment with someone they can rely on for understanding and care in times of distress. Caring for a traumatized child is stressful; as this book attests, our best resource for coping with stress is secure attachment. To provide support, you need support—personal and perhaps professional. You need specialized knowledge. But most important, like the therapists who provide effective trauma treatment, you will rely on your *skill in being human*. We all have this skill, which enables us to feel connected with others, in joy and in pain. But we need a high level of skill in feeling connected with traumatic levels of emotional pain, and we need help in refining our natural skill.

You have found a reliable guide.

JON G. ALLEN, PhD
Menninger Department of Psychiatry
and Behavioral Sciences
Baylor College of Medicine

Acknowledgments

Writing this book has been a labor of love, and it has only come to fruition thanks to support and guidance from some very special people.

First and foremost, thank you to Kitty Moore and Christine Benton, editors extraordinaire. Your warm encouragement and enthusiasm for this book combined with your insightful feedback helped turn my jumbled thoughts into a precise and well-ordered work of literature. I will be forever grateful for your handholding and expert guidance as we crafted the manuscript, and always appreciated the excitement, wisdom, and humorous spirit you both exuded in our interactions.

Next, I have been incredibly blessed with a series of mentors throughout my career. This book would not exist without their supportive and skillful guidance. Most central to this book are Liz Newlin, who so clearly articulated to me the important role of the family in healing from trauma, and Jon Allen, whose way of opening our mentalizing group has formed the foundation of everything I believe about therapy and healing. Many thanks to Ron Acierno, Patty Daza, George Bombel, Chris Fowler, Colleen O'Byrne, Marcia Laviage, Lawrence Thompson Jr., Claudia Mustafa, Sara May, Kim Pfaff, Marcela Torres, Leigh Baker, and Drew Westen for your support throughout my career and for inspiring me to pursue a career in the treatment of trauma.

Many thanks to Mollie Gordon and Phuong Nguyen for your support in the curriculum adaptation process—I am so happy to have you both in my corner.

To my colleagues, whom I am lucky enough to call dear friends:

Thank you. Adelia Sabinstev, you are the warmest, most supportive person I've met. Thank you for your ongoing backing, and for your expert consultation that helped me flesh out Chapter 9. Also, many thanks to Emily Roth Van Laan, Lindsey Hogan, Brittany Lawnin, Rose Yang, Jenny Hughes, and Janelle Veenstra for your friendship and psychological insights.

Many thanks to fellow author Ashley Winstead, for your publishing guidance and cheerleading.

Thank you to Kathryn Kase, whose thoughtful questions inspired me to think about the role parents can play in healing and recovery.

To my oldest friends: Thank you to Sharone Tobias, for two and a half decades of dreaming big and for the tough love necessary to make it through writing a book. Also to Robyn Munn, for your "darling" writing advice.

Because this book was written amid school shutdowns, a pregnancy, and early postpartum days, thank you to the amazing "pod" of school teachers, babysitters, mom friends, and caregivers who helped support our family in this time, especially to Amanda Moon Lee, Joy Jacobson, Lachelle Henton, Jamie Wilkinson, Jenn Char, and Jasmin Prince.

Thank you to my mother, Carol Goldberg, for consistently being available and reliable, and for constantly pushing me forward, and my father, Michael Goldberg, who always believed I could do anything.

To my children, Sophie and Franklin; you are my everything. Connecting with you both has brought to life all I believed about attachment, and our quality time fueled me up and kept me going through long nights of writing.

And finally, to my husband, Evan Mintz. I didn't know how right I was when I quoted Freud at our wedding, "How bold one gets when one is sure of being loved." There's no chance I would have been so daring as to write a book without your emotional support and technical writing assistance. All of the great one-liners and pop culture references in this book are from your incredible mind. I don't know how I got lucky enough to marry you.

Has Your Child Been Traumatized?

Introduction

Let me tell you a story about one of the unluckiest patients I have ever met, a twelve-year-old boy named Rick. Many studies over the last few decades have found that nearly two-thirds of all people experience at least one adverse event during childhood, but this boy had lived through more than most. When he was a baby, Rick's family was forced to flee New Orleans when their home was destroyed by Hurricane Katrina. Years later, after his family had gotten back on their feet in Houston, Hurricane Harvey struck and engulfed everything they owned in a devastating flood. At his new school, he had his nose broken when a bully punched him in the face. Finally, after all of this, as he was on his way to see me for our first therapy session, his mother's car was T-boned by a truck. It seemed like this poor kid could not catch a break.

I was early in my career when I first read Rick's referral form and felt ill equipped to help someone who had gone through so much. Yet I was shocked when we first met. His energetic, upbeat demeanor and goofy sense of humor seemed so out of place with what he had endured. Sure, he looked worn out and on edge when describing the hurricane-related nightmares he suffered on a regular basis, and he scored in the clinically significant range on a test for posttraumatic stress that I administered. But he seemed to be doing so well in the rest of his life. He was excelling in school, described healthy relationships with his friends, and remained unexpectedly optimistic about his future.

Rick's perplexing condition finally made sense to me when his mother joined us at the end of the first session. His face immediately lit up as he began telling me about their mother–son plans to go play mini-golf after every session. His mom joined in, explaining that mini-golf was their "thing." As I got to know the duo better, it became apparent that her parenting practices may have helped her son begin to heal before he even set foot in my office. After a few months of work with Rick on trauma-focused therapy and with his mother on some practical trauma-based parenting skills, his nightmares and other posttraumatic stress symptoms had practically disappeared. Years later, I smiled when I heard he had received a merit-based scholarship to a wonderful state university and was continuing to make his mother proud.

What I hope you take from this story is the importance of the parent–child relationship, especially in healing from trauma. I would even go so far as to say a warm, nurturing relationship with a skilled caregiver is more valuable to a child's recovery than weekly therapy sessions with the most knowledgeable therapist in the world. In other words, *you* are the key to helping your child heal from and thrive after trauma.

This can sound like a heavy responsibility—you have the weight of a child's future resting on your shoulders. Don't worry! Parenting a traumatized child doesn't require therapist-level skills, sage-like wisdom, or supernatural levels of strength and patience. In fact, everything you need is inside you right now. The skills necessary to care for a child who has experienced an adverse event flow naturally from the parenting abilities and love that you already possess. This book will provide specific insights into how trauma works and show you how to channel your instinct to nurture into effective support and healing.

I first became interested in the role of parents in helping children heal while working as a therapist as part of a clinical trial for trauma-focused cognitive-behavioral therapy (TF-CBT), a gold-standard approach to treating trauma in children. While I observed many of the children I worked with experience a significant reduction in posttraumatic stress symptoms, the kids who improved the most and in the shortest amount of time were those who had incredibly supportive, engaged parents or other caregivers. Having worked with this type of patient for a decade, I've come to the conclusion that therapy is sometimes necessary yet often not sufficient to fully treat child trauma. On the other hand, a strong caregiver–child relationship is often necessary, and sometimes sufficient to facilitate healing.

You may be confused about whether your child has been traumatized after being exposed to an event that left them emotionally distressed or physically harmed in some way. Or perhaps you know your child needs some support, but you're not sure where to start. Maybe your child is exhibiting troubling behavioral changes—increase in aggression, lack of interest in spending time with friends, falling grades—and you're not sure how to make sense of them. Or perhaps your child is experiencing panic, stress, or frequent intense reminders of the event and you feel powerless to help in these acute moments of vulnerability.

The goal of this book is to help you make sense of what has happened to your child and what she is experiencing after a potentially traumatic event and then empower you to assist your child in moving through it.

What to Expect from This Book

Overall, this book can help you if you think your child has experienced a potentially traumatic event and you're not sure what to do next. You're probably asking yourself questions like:

- Will my child be okay? Or forever scarred by this experience?
- How do children become traumatized?
- What is posttraumatic stress disorder (PTSD)?

- Why is my child acting differently than other kids who had a similar experience?
- What can I do to help?

These are all perfectly normal questions to have. Children have their own internal lives that even they themselves struggle to understand, let alone articulate to others—and things become even more difficult as kids turn into teenagers. That's why, throughout the book, I try to make things as easy as possible for you to sort out by including illustrations and anecdotes from my practice that can help you understand important matters such as when a child's reaction to a potentially traumatic event is cause for concern and when professional help is necessary.

In the aftermath of an adverse event, you'll be able to provide the support your child needs, starting with building a foundation for healing and helping your child build a buffer against future traumatic stress. You'll learn skills that will help you:

- Respond to trauma triggers
- Make sense of confusing and troubling new behaviors, like increased tearfulness
- Set and enforce rules with a traumatized child
- Recognize and deal with avoidance
- Address the trauma-related problems common to teenagers, including dangerous impulsive behaviors
- Prevent a resurgence of trauma symptoms later in your child's life

This book is made up of twelve chapters that will guide you in parenting your child after exposure to a potentially traumatic event. The first chapters provide an overview of trauma and will help you make sense of the confusing days, weeks, and months after a potentially traumatic experience. In the aftermath of a scary incident, it can be hard to tease apart whether or not a child has been traumatized. You will also come to understand why some children develop trauma responses and others do not and how to differentiate between healthy and more concerning behavior. And finally, after understanding these foundational issues of trauma and traumatic responses, you will revisit the overarching idea that a strong parent–child relationship is one of the most important factors in helping your child build a resilient response in the face of adversity. You will even learn concrete, easy-to-implement skills that can deepen the parent–child relationship and facilitate the healing process.

Next I'll describe the behavioral changes often seen in children following a potentially traumatic event. Some of these behaviors are common in young children; others are more specifically seen in older adolescents. Anecdotes and illustrations based on composites of the children I've treated will help you understand what you might see in your child following a potentially traumatic experience. This includes trauma triggers, or stimuli that pop up and remind your child of their scary experience, as well as increased emotionality, minor misbehavior, avoidance, major misbehavior, self-harm, and impulsive behaviors. Skills taught in the third part of the book will help you handle these confusing, sometimes troubling behaviors to help your child heal.

While the parent–child relationship is the single most critical factor in facilitating healing after a traumatic event, sometimes professional help is recommended. That is why this book also provides an overview of different types of therapy available. In Chapter 11 I lay out a structured approach to identifying a practitioner who might be a good fit for your child or family—or even for you.

The final chapter will help you anticipate any future speed bumps your child may encounter over the course of life. Many children and adolescents who have experienced potentially traumatic events go on to lead healthy, productive lives, seemingly unencumbered by their adverse experience. While they can certainly thrive, even traumatized children who have been treated successfully may experience a resurgence of symptoms at later points in life. By anticipating this possible resurgence, you can help build your child's confidence and ensure they know what to do if symptoms ever return.

Armed with the knowledge and skills provided in this book, you will be able to confidently guide your child through the healing process toward a healthy, happy future.

PART I

Understanding Trauma

1

What Is Trauma?

Whenever I drive to work, my commute takes me past a strip mall along the freeway that has a Chinese restaurant, a popcorn store, and a small medical office called "24-Hour Trauma Center."

That name always makes me think, because when most people talk about the trauma in their lives, they're not describing the sorts of things that land them in the emergency room. Maybe it's two best friends in high school commiserating about a chemistry midterm that was "traumatic." Or maybe it's a newly married woman talking about how Thanksgiving dinner with the in-laws was "completely traumatizing." Or maybe it's coworkers talking about how they were "totally traumatized" by the shocking finale of their favorite streamed TV series.

The "trauma" people usually talk about is more likely to have them texting friends to vent than rushing to the strip mall doctor for medical help.

As a psychologist, I work with people who talk about their trauma. While their experiences may not require the stitches and antibiotics offered by a medical doctor, they do require a different kind of medical attention. In the field of mental health, however, trauma has a specific meaning. It's not the injury to living tissue, as physicians use the term. Nor does it refer to the everyday uncomfortable experiences that people like to rant about with friends.

For psychologists and therapists, trauma is a biological, psychological, and social reaction to an event that was genuinely frightening.

This trauma has observable and describable effects on people, often labeled as a "trauma response." These responses can look different depending on the person, but they usually fall into a few categories. They can include intrusive memories of the event, nightmares, and flashbacks; changes in arousal such as an increased startle response and difficulty with concentration; avoidance of people, places, and things that can remind one of the trauma; and increased negative thoughts and feelings about oneself and the world.

In the field of mental health, *trauma* isn't a word thrown around cavalierly. It is a condition that should be taken seriously. If left unaddressed, it can impair people's lives. And if handled properly, it can be healed—and sometimes even leave people stronger and more empowered.

Types of Incidents That Can Cause Trauma

So where does trauma come from? What "counts" as a traumatic experience?

Almost any frightening experience can be traumatic. It all depends on how someone reacts over time. However, mental health experts have found that certain types of events can routinely elicit trauma responses—especially in a child.

The most common potentially traumatic events include being exposed to actual or threatened death, serious injury, or sexual violation. This doesn't mean a person has to be physically hurt or otherwise impacted personally. Witnessing one of these terrible experiences inflicted on someone else can be enough to result in trauma. Even learning about the experience after the fact and knowing it hurt someone you care about or depend on can induce trauma, especially if there is repeated or extreme exposure to aversive details.

One of the more routine causes of trauma in my practice as a psychologist is car crashes. A child can be traumatized after being in a scary wreck. Some children also develop a trauma response after learning that one of their parents was hurt in a serious collision. Even seeing a car crash happen while playing at the park can be traumatic for a child, particularly if something about the event is especially shocking, violent, or gruesome. After any one of these scenarios, it would be perfectly normal for a child to have trouble sleeping or try to avoid riding in cars. However, these symptoms typically fade as part of the routine healing process. When the symptoms don't resolve, or maybe even get worse, we can confidently say that a child has been traumatized. The child was exposed to threatened death or serious injury, had a trauma response, and it interfered with the child's day-to-day life.

That's trauma.

Adverse Childhood Experiences

Childhood trauma may sound intimidating, but in reality almost every child can overcome a potentially traumatic event. In fact, **most children who undergo potentially traumatic experiences get better without needing any professional help**. The trauma responses decline naturally over time. Those nightmares after the car crash go away on their own without any professional intervention.

Unfortunately, that's not always what happens. In the worst-case scenarios, traumatic events cause children to experience so much stress that it inflicts long-term harm to their physical health.

In the mid-1990s, a study conducted by the Centers for Disease Control and Prevention (CDC) and Kaiser Permanente surveyed over seventeen thousand HMO members and found that certain incidents during youth could have lifelong implications for physical and mental health. The researchers referred to these potentially traumatic experiences as "adverse childhood experiences," or ACEs. The ACEs identified by this study and others are listed in the box on pages 12–13. These extensive (but not all-inclusive) lists show that potentially traumatic events are not a cut-and-dried, black-and-white phenomenon.

Potentially Traumatic Events Found
in Research and Clinical Practice

The CDC–Kaiser study identified these events that can be traumatizing:

- Physical abuse
- Verbal abuse
- Sexual abuse
- Physical neglect
- Emotional neglect
- Having a parent with a substance abuse problem
- Witnessing domestic violence
- Having a family member in prison
- Having a family member with mental illness
- Separation from a parent due to separation, divorce, or abandonment

These events were selected because they were prevalent in the people studied, but additional adverse experiences have been identified by other research:

- Bullying
- Motor vehicle accidents
- Sudden, unexpected, or shocking loss of a loved one
- Having a sibling with a substance abuse problem
- Sexual violence in a dating relationship
- Emotional abuse in a dating relationship
- Homelessness
- Events that took place in refugee camps or wartime
- Natural disasters
- School shootings

- Mass shootings outside of school
- Witnessing community violence
- Medical trauma

In my practice, I've also seen idiosyncratic traumas stem from events that are less represented in the research but can be just as terrifying. These include:

- Being attacked by the family pet
- Being thrown into a pool or other body of water and not knowing how to swim
- Exposure to pornography or other age-inappropriate violent content via elder siblings or neighbors
- Being trapped by oneself (locked in a room, stuck in an elevator)
- Being left with a caregiver who is essentially a stranger for an undetermined period of time
- Being forced to kneel on rice or other corporal punishment for bad behavior

Any event that is frightening, dangerous, or violent or poses a threat to the child's life or bodily integrity, or even a loved one's life or bodily integrity, can be experienced as traumatic.

The researchers found that exposure to these experiences put children at a higher lifetime risk for psychological issues including depression and suicide attempts, social issues including failure to complete schooling and increased rates of high-risk sexual behaviors, and even medical problems such as diabetes and heart disease. The research done to date serves as a reminder of the powerful impact that trauma and ACEs can have on a child's life.

This information may seem overwhelming at first for anyone

invested in a child's well-being. But it is specifically because the stakes could be so high that it's important to respond diligently when a child endures a potentially traumatic event and ensure the child gets the right kind of support. Throughout this book, I'll describe what that support looks like and offer strategies on the best ways to deliver it, so that you can help your child avoid these worst-case outcomes.

Why Adverse Childhood Events Can Be Traumatic

There used to be a Sunday morning kids' show on local television networks called *Wonderama*. After three hours of kids dancing, playing, and doing sketch comedy, the host, Bob McAllister, would close out each episode by singing a song, "Kids Are People Too."

"We may be young, and not full grown / But we have problems of our own," McAllister would sing, joined by kids in the audience. He may not have been a psychologist, but the Baltimore TV host had latched on to an important aspect of childhood mental health—it can be hard to be a kid!

"It isn't easy going all day / winning and losing in the games that we play / doing our homework, learning in school / and trying to live by the Golden Rule."

Through the eyes of an adult, kids seem to have it easy. They don't need to go to work or have bills to pay or much in the way of responsibility. But to a kid, that lack of responsibility can feel more like a lack of structure. The world is vast and confusing, and kids don't fully understand how it works. Each day is spent gaining new experiences and trying to piece together a rough comprehension of how everything operates. As children learn and grow, they form different beliefs about how things should function—their own mental ordering of the world. In the field of mental health, we call these beliefs *schemas*.

Imagine a toddler seeing a kitten for the first time. It's small, fluffy, and has four legs and a tail. That's a kitten. When the child later sees a puppy for the first time—or any other small, fluffy animal with four legs and a tail—she may shout out "kitten!" After all, it fits her schema of what a kitten is. After being corrected and informed about the difference between a puppy and a kitten, the child will eventually update her schemas and build a new, more nuanced understanding of the world.

Starting with his 1967 book *The Diagnosis and Management of Depression*, Dr. Aaron Beck helped therapists grasp how schemas can impact mental health. Schemas aren't just how we understand what things are, but also how we make sense of the world around us. These concepts aren't usually referenced aloud but nonetheless remain deeply ingrained in our minds: Parents are caring. The world is a safe and fair place. Good things happen to good people, and bad things happen to bad people.

Many of us hold on to these schemas throughout our lives. They serve us effectively when they help us make sense of how the world works—or at least should work. However, sometimes reality comes into conflict with these schemas. That can be a challenging experience for even the most mature adult. For children, it can be devastating.

I regularly see patients who have just endured traumas so impactful that they're driven to revise their schemas—maybe the world isn't so safe after all.

Consider the experience of a ten-year-old boy who just said goodbye to his mom as she walked out the door to run some errands. She runs errands all the time. Nothing bad ever happens. He has no reason to fear some nefarious force would intervene and send harm her way. But then, one rainy evening, she is hit by a car skidding on slick asphalt in the grocery store parking lot. The injury sends her to the hospital but inflicts no long-term medical harm. The son, however, suddenly finds his assumptions about the world brought into question. The errands actually aren't so safe. It turns out the world may be a very, very dangerous place.

Driven by this revised schema, the ten-year-old boy may start acting and feeling differently. Mom's regular errands will spark fear in him, and he'll beg her not to leave the house. Maybe rain and thunder are viewed as legitimate threats rather than routine weather, and he will stay inside instead of joining his friends jumping in puddles. His schemas change, interfering with his ability to live a normal life. That's the trauma starting to manifest itself.

Avoidance: A Coping Strategy and a Mechanism for the Development of Trauma

Children sometimes cope with fear-based schemas by practicing avoidance behaviors that can help lessen their anxieties. In other words, the ten-year-old may try his hardest to convince his mom not to run errands long after she has healed so that he doesn't have to grapple with the potential dangers that lurk beyond the front door. This strategy may make sense in the short term, but it undermines natural recovery. The more a child tries to avoid the people, places, things, and situations that cause distress, the bigger and scarier they become.

A helpful metaphor I use to educate patients about the role of avoidance in posttraumatic stress is that of the anxiety tiger, originally developed by Steven Hayes in his 2005 book *Get Out of Your Mind and Into Your Life*. Imagine you are lounging on your sofa, minding your own business, when you notice a tiny tiger cub outside, mewling at you. He looks hungry. He is cute but also a little bit scary, and you'd prefer to get back to lounging. You recall you have a hunk of meat in your fridge, and without thinking, you grab it and toss it out your open door, and the cub follows and leaves your house. Problem solved.

But the next day, the cub returns. He's a little bit bigger, probably because you fed him that delicious meat, and a little bit scarier. Accordingly, you feel a bit more anxious, and more motivated to get this tiger out of your living room. You do have more meat in the fridge, so like yesterday, you grab it and toss it out the door. The cub follows, and your stress levels fall. What a relief that you can so easily solve this problem.

Until the next day. You know the drill. The pattern repeats, day in and day out, until you have a full-grown tiger staring you down.

In this metaphor, the tossing of the meat is akin to the practice of avoidance when thinking about or encountering stimuli that remind you of the scary event. To go back to our hypothetical about the ten-year-old and his mother, if he had been able to dissuade her from running errands for three months and then she got fed up with this practice and suddenly decided to push back, you can bet this boy would feel like a fully grown tiger was staring him down.

While many factors can influence whether a child becomes traumatized or goes on to heal after a frightening event, avoidance frequently plays a large role in bridging the gap between an adverse experience and the development of a more long-standing trauma response.

Common Misconceptions about Trauma

Now that you know a bit about trauma, ACEs, and their relation to each other, let's cover some common misconceptions.

"This Hardly Ever Happens to Kids"

Parents are shocked when I explain that almost two out of three of the people in the United States have had exposure to at least one adverse childhood experience. People often overestimate how happy and well-adjusted others are, which can make us feel isolated and hopeless when struggling with our own stressors. The reality is more in line with the common adage "We all have a cross to bear."

This isn't just anecdotal. In the original CDC–Kaiser study, more than half of respondents said they had experienced at least one adverse experience while growing up. One in six had had four or more such experiences. More recent research on the same topic has revealed similar prevalence rates. A 2018 study published by the American Medical Association surveyed close to 250,000 adults and found that 61.55% of respondents had experienced at least one adverse childhood experience. As in the original ACE study, about one-quarter of subjects reported exposure to four or more ACEs. With the increase in stressors related to the global COVID-19 pandemic that swept the world in 2020 and beyond, you can bet those rates will soar even higher for children growing up today.

Even after learning about the prevalence of ACEs, parents and children alike are surprised to discover that their specific scary experience is also incredibly common. People of all ages who face trauma often express a sense of shame around their experience and their response to it. This shame can make people feel alone in their struggle. So it can be helpful to keep in mind that all types of ACEs are fairly common and that your child has a community of peers who have gone through the same thing. The box on the facing page shows prevalence rates for the six most commonly reported ACEs, from the original mid-1990s data and more recent data, reported from 2018 onward.

Though rates for specific traumas have risen and fallen over time, it appears overall rates of exposure to ACEs remain incredibly high.

Adverse experiences are, for the time being, an unfortunate and often inevitable part of life. However, these high prevalence rates also mean that children are not alone in their ordeals. Furthermore, the pervasiveness of adverse experiences lends itself to an extensive research base, which shows that the majority of children do go on to heal and thrive after an adverse experience. For more information on this, see Chapter 2.

"This Experience Will Leave My Child Permanently Damaged"

Another common misconception I come across is the fear parents have about their child being scarred forever in some way by exposure to a potentially traumatic event.

Prevalence of the Most Common Adverse Childhood Events

Adverse childhood event	CDC–Kaiser ACE prevalence rates (1995–1997)	Updated prevalence rates (2018–2020)
Sexual abuse	24.7% (f)* 16% (m)	25–33% (f) 12.5% (m)
Physical abuse	27% (f) 29.9% (m)	17.53% (f) 18.38% (m)
Emotional abuse	13.1% (f) 7.6% (m)	33.94% (f) 34.92% (m)
Household substance abuse	29.5% (f) 23.8% (m)	26.33% (f) 28.72% (m)
Household mental illness	23.3% (f) 14.8% (m)	19.19% (f) 13.71% (m)
Parental separation or divorce	24.5% (f) 21.8% (m)	27.80% (f) 27.45% (m)

*(f) stands for female-identifying respondents, (m) for male. Percentages reflect segments of the sample that experienced the specific event (e.g., 24.7% of female-identifying respondents sampled in the original CDC-Kaiser study endorsed experiencing sexual abuse, the remaining 75.3% denied experiencing this).

Here's what I say to that: While children will likely always remember the scary thing that happened to them, it does not mean they can't go on to lead a life just as successful, happy, and adaptive as the life they were destined for pre–adverse event.

German philosopher Friedrich Nietzsche famously wrote, "What does not kill me makes me stronger." While I would argue that this is not always true for everyone who experiences an adverse event, there is a growing body of literature on the psychological concept of post-traumatic growth. This idea was developed by psychologists Richard Tedeschi and Lawrence Calhoun in the mid-1990s and is defined as positive, meaningful psychological changes that an individual can experience after enduring a potentially traumatic event. It might look like an increased appreciation for life, spiritual changes, a greater sense of personal strength and new possibilities in life, or a renewed capacity for relationships.

While I don't frequently see major, life-changing epiphanies or other dramatic shifts in personality or outlook on life after an adverse experience occurs, what I have seen more often is improved relationships between parent and child at the conclusion of treatment. Many children have remarked after the end of therapy that they feel they can turn to their parents in times of distress as a source of support.

Trauma can and does regularly have lifelong negative impacts on social, psychological, and medical health outcomes. The biggest risk for these outcomes is living in a family where the child is not supported or believed, where the child's feelings are belittled or dismissed, or where the child is met with parental apathy. But if parents can learn to be supportive and skillful amid the chaos of trauma, they may just find their child in a healthier place than before the adverse event.

"All Children Need Help after an Adverse Experience"

One final common misconception I frequently hear about trauma comes from well-meaning type-A parents. Several times a year, I see parents who bring their child to therapy after an adverse event, and I meet a happy, well-adjusted child who denies all trauma symptoms. These parents do not always believe me when I tell them their child is fine and has no need for treatment—they're convinced that their child needs help after experiencing something scary.

"But he was so jumpy the next day!" "Are you sure? She had

nightmares three nights in a row right after it happened!" "But how can a kid be okay after experiencing something like that?" These are all common retorts I encounter when trying to reassure these worried parents. Take comfort in knowing that displaying some stress symptoms immediately following a scary event is a healthy part of the healing process, and the fact that an event sounds terrifying doesn't mean your child personally perceived it in that way.

How Does a Child End Up Traumatized by an Event?

As you now know, many children experience adverse events. While many exhibit symptoms immediately following the event, these symptoms often fade naturally in the following days and weeks. In some children, however, these symptoms do not naturally fade and may even grow in intensity.

But why might one child develop trauma while another goes on to heal naturally?

I've already noted that avoidance plays a large role in the development of trauma symptoms, but there are many additional factors that impact this puzzling equation. When trying to determine where this difference comes from, I always like to start by looking at the small, idiosyncratic variances in the way children experience the event.

Minor Differences in How Children Experience the Event

Patty and Elena are best friends in their third-grade classroom. Both girls are well adjusted and come from loving homes. One ordinary Wednesday, while sitting in science class, they hear a series of loud pops resembling gunshots. Their school reacts appropriately and places their classroom in lockdown. Patty and Elena are hiding behind different desks, at opposite ends of the room. Patty has the good fortune of being next to her teacher, who is a calming presence. Elena is crouched next to Ethan, the youngest of four boys, who tells her that his older brothers told him about school shootings and that they were all going to die. It turns out the loud bangs were a couple of truant teenagers setting off fireworks down the street and no one was ever in any danger. After school that day, Patty recalled the events to her parents and sounded excited to be telling them about something novel. Elena, however, went on to develop ongoing nightmares and now throws tantrums every morning in a bid to avoid school.

In this scenario, both Patty and Elena experienced the same potentially traumatic event. Patty experienced it as something strange, but not threatening. Elena got the message that her life was in danger.

The Child's Age

Chronological and developmental age can also have a significant impact on whether an adverse event becomes a trauma.

For example, in very young children (up to age two), trauma responses are often partially dictated by how their primary caregivers respond to the potentially traumatic event. Depending on the type of adverse event, you may have more or less control over this. If you are physically okay and can remain calm and give your baby comfort or keep your toddler close, you probably won't see too many trauma symptoms. On the other hand, if the adverse event caused you to be hospitalized and separated from your very young child for an extended period of time, this might be incredibly disturbing to the child. Additionally, in contrast to older children, very young children are more likely to be traumatized by something scary happening to a primary caregiver and less likely to be traumatized by something happening directly to them, provided their caregiver can respond in a calm, loving way (again, this is not always possible, depending on the severity of the event).

If something scary happened to your family and you did not respond calmly, please do not fret. Every parent has been there. It is terrifying to think of something bad happening to your child, especially a very young one you still see as a fragile little baby—even the first scraped knee or bloody lip can send a parent into full-blown freak-out mode.

Risk and Protective Factors

It's easy to understand how, as in the story of Patty and Elena, two kids sitting in two different places can have varying responses to the same potentially traumatic event. But what if they had been sitting next to each other and both heard Ethan's panicked response? They could still have two entirely different experiences of the event. In other words, there are many factors that can help predict how a child will respond to trauma.

In the field of psychology, we often think of risk and protective factors as constructs that make an individual more or less vulnerable to the development of a psychological disorder. While we can't run from our genetic makeup or our exposure to an adverse event, certain other factors can affect the likelihood that a child will become traumatized following such an event.

Family Trauma History

Scientists have found that a familial history of trauma can have an intergenerational effect. Extensive research has been conducted with the children and grandchildren of survivors of the Holocaust and genocides in Rwanda, Nigeria, Cambodia, Armenia, and the former Yugoslavia. Studies have revealed increased rates of numerous mental health disorders, including PTSD, in the offspring of survivors. Specific symptoms include a distrust of the world, an ever-present sense of danger, and separation anxiety.

There are many different theories out there about why this happens. Many believe the intergenerational trauma stems at least in part from a biological mechanism. Survivors' experiences result in a permanently raised level of cortisol—a stress hormone—which then gets passed through the generations.

There are also psychological components that contribute to this phenomenon. Rachel Dekel and Hadass Goldblatt, two psychologists studying intergenerational transmission of trauma, explain these factors in a 2008 review paper, "Is There Intergenerational Transmission of Trauma?" Literature they reviewed hypothesized that parents with PTSD have difficulty coping with uncomfortable emotions. In attempts to alleviate their emotional pain, they may project their feelings of aggression, shame, and guilt onto their children. Their children then may go on to identify with those experiences, feeling guilty and ashamed. If a child is already feeling this way *before* the occurrence of an adverse event, you can bet that child will be especially vulnerable to the development of more intense trauma symptoms.

At the same time, parents who survive these horrific events with resilience may actually pass those *positive* traits on to the next generations. Luciana Braga, Marcelo Mello, and Jose Fiks, researchers at the Sao Paulo School of Medicine, conducted interviews with Brazilian offspring of Holocaust survivors in 2012. They found that survivors who coped well with their trauma had children and grandchildren who demonstrated similar patterns of resilience.

Temperament

In the study of child development, temperament is thought of as a child's innate way of being, which later develops into a personality. It is heritable, observable in early life, and stable as people age. What was your son like before the adverse event? Did he display a tendency to get upset intensely and easily? If so, he might be a bit more vulnerable to the development of stress symptoms. Perhaps your daughter was easygoing and unfazed by major adjustments. If that is the case, her temperament could be a protective factor against trauma.

Coping Skills

Stress is an inevitable part of life. What does your child look like when experiencing normal, day-to-day stressors? If your son feels frustrated that his little sister has stolen his toy, does he have a meltdown and try to attack her? If so, he might be more vulnerable to the development of posttraumatic stress following a stressor. But if your child is instead able to use his words, take some deep breaths, or turn to a caregiver for help, great news—these skills can be a buffer against the development of trauma.

Role Models

Our children know that the grown-ups in their lives also go through stressful situations. When they see you dealing with pressure from a work deadline or some other routine stressor, what are they observing about how you cope with stress? Seeing you talking about your feelings, getting support, exercising, or counting to ten will go a long way in teaching them how to respond to their own stressors. There is a saying in my field, "We do what we know." In this context, this means children will imitate the coping they see in their models. At the same time, a child who sees a caregiver modeling poor coping can't be expected to know what to do upon encountering a mundane stressor, much less a potentially traumatic event.

Stable Living Environment

After an adverse event, children can feel like their lives are spinning out of control. Knowing that they have a consistent caregiver in a stable home can go a long way in grounding them. At the same time, bouncing around between caregivers, whether foster homes or several different biological relatives, can be unmooring to a child. After experiencing a traumatic event, this instability can be especially unsettling.

Meaningful Social Support

Does your young child have an especially close relationship with Grandma? Does your preteen have a close circle of friends? Having people they feel like they can turn to in times of distress is one of the biggest protective factors children can have and a parent can hope for. Inversely, children who feel like they don't have anyone they can share their big feelings with after a scary event are more vulnerable to the development of posttraumatic stress. Think about it this way: Whenever you're struggling with something, which times feel more overwhelming—the times you are able to chat about it with a trusted friend or loved one or the times you feel all alone with it?

Community Support and Involvement

A sense of belonging can go a long way in protecting a child against the development of trauma. Are there local community centers where your child is known? Does your son or daughter play for a community sports team or take an art class at the rec center? If so, this could also help protect your child from developing a trauma response. At the same time, a lack of connection to their surroundings might make children more vulnerable.

Severity and Duration of the Event

A child who experiences an adverse event that is ongoing and more intense in nature will be more vulnerable to the development of trauma than a child who experiences a shorter, milder adverse event. Compare a child who is bullied every single day of the school year, is routinely beaten up and left with bruises, and was thrown into a garbage can to a child who was bullied by being pushed up against a wall and threatened one time. Both examples are undoubtedly scary, but the child who endures routine and more severe bullying may be more likely to have the worse outcome, all other risk and protective factors being equal.

Parental Support

When your child comes to you with something troubling, listen patiently and determine together how you can best support the child. This will go a long way in buffering your child from some of the harmful effects of adverse childhood events. As we will expand on in Chapter 3, a strong, supportive parent–child relationship is one of the most crucial protective factors against posttraumatic stress.

The first step in helping your child heal after a potentially traumatic experience is to have a basic understanding of adverse events and trauma. I hope after reading this chapter you feel more informed about what trauma is, how it differs from adverse experiences, and why some children may go on to develop trauma while others are fine. I also hope you now understand that exposure to potentially traumatic events is incredibly common and your child can still go on to thrive. The next chapter will help you take a closer look at your own child to determine whether the child has been traumatized and to what extent so you can know how to proceed in the most helpful way.

2

Has Your Child Been Traumatized?

In the aftermath of a scary experience, it can be hard to tease apart whether a child has been traumatized. Some parents may assume their typically moody twelve-year-old was doing just fine after losing the family home in a fire because the only behavioral change they noticed was his seeming a bit more reserved. In reality, this boy may be suffering in silence. Likewise, a parent might assume something is seriously wrong with a younger child who has had nightmares and sleep avoidance in the week following a car crash, when these types of symptoms can be perfectly normal and not a sign of any mental health issues following a potentially traumatic experience. This chapter will help you make sense of the confusing days, weeks, and months following a potentially traumatic event so you can better understand what your child may be experiencing.

The Trajectory of Posttraumatic Stress

Each child may be unique, but after a potentially traumatic experience people often follow similar patterns of behavior. Understanding these patterns can help you understand what your child is going through, why the child is acting in certain ways, and what you can do to help.

Adults suffering from posttraumatic stress typically follow one of four key trajectories: resilience, recovery, delayed symptoms, and chronic symptoms.

- *Resilient trajectory:* Individuals experience mild or nonexistent symptoms after the exposure to a potentially traumatic event, and the mild symptoms resolve quickly.
- *Recovery trajectory:* Individuals initially experience significant levels of acute symptoms (those that appear suddenly and are relatively severe) but experience gradual recovery.
- *Delayed symptom trajectory:* Individuals experience low levels of acute symptoms immediately following the exposure but over time have worsening posttraumatic stress symptoms.
- *Chronic symptom trajectory:* Individuals experience high levels of both acute and ongoing symptoms.

These trajectories are a relatively new discovery in the field of mental health, having been classified in adults in 2004 by psychologist George Bonanno in his article "Loss, Trauma, and Human Resilience: Have We Underestimated the Human Capacity to Thrive after Extremely Aversive Events?"

However, kids aren't adults, and several studies have found that children don't adhere to these *exact* same paths. Most of this research has found that children tend to follow only three of the previously identified trajectories: resilient, recovery, and chronic.

One such study, conducted by Robyne Le Brocque and colleagues at the University of Queensland in 2010, followed children ages six to sixteen who had accidental injuries. The majority of the kids fell along the resilient path. They had minimal stress symptoms after their injuries and hospital admission. One-third followed the recovery trajectory and suffered from significant posttraumatic stress symptoms that eventually receded in the subsequent months. Finally, a small sliver—only 10 percent—qualified as having chronic symptoms and demonstrated continuous posttraumatic stress even months later.

Subsequent research identified the same three trajectories in other types of potentially traumatic events, including natural disasters. In contrast to adults, most of these studies did not find a group of kids who had a delayed onset of symptoms. (A small number of studies have found some children experience a delayed onset of trauma symptoms, but even in these studies, few children fell into this category compared to other groups.)

There is no research yet that explains this discrepancy between adults and children, but as a therapist I can say that kids—especially young kids—often show their struggles on the surface. Their defense mechanisms are not always as evolved and ingrained as those of adults, who may be masters at pushing down their own painful thoughts and feelings. In a way that makes your job easier—there are fewer worries about ticking time bombs of posttraumatic stress in the weeks ahead.

Overall, this research offers a few key lessons for caregivers.

First, kids are more resilient than you think. Many symptoms that occur after adverse events will often lessen naturally over time without any professional intervention. Second, most kids who do experience stress after an adverse event routinely recover gradually and return to their pre-event levels of healthy functioning. These kids could benefit from some supportive therapy but aren't in dire need of it. Finally, some kids will experience chronic stress and do absolutely require professional help. There is nothing wrong with needing or getting this care. A child who falls into this category isn't any less strong, smart, or capable than her peers. Whether due to genetics, the specific circumstances of the trauma, or the litany of other risk and protective factors discussed in Chapter 1, these children would certainly benefit from directive trauma-focused interventions from a therapist. However, no matter which trajectory your child follows, the skills and concepts in this book will help you support your child to heal.

So what does each trajectory look like in reality?

Kids who go through the same traumatic experience can end up following different paths. Consider the following example:

Kenny, Sebastian, Brian, and Marcus were best friends who had just finished sixth grade together. Before going their separate ways over the summer, they each write in the others' yearbooks about how seventh grade is going to be the best year ever. Just before the beginning of the school year, however, Marcus dies by suicide. Kenny, Sebastian, and Brian, who had not kept in touch over the three-month break, were each shocked by their friend's death. To support the students, the school sent a psychologist to meet with each of the three friends.

Kenny: Resilient Group

When Kenny's mother told him about Marcus's death, he refused to believe her and remarked several times that she was telling some sort of "sick joke." It took a few hours for him to come to terms with the sad reality of the moment. In his meetings with the school psychologist, Kenny shared some feelings of shock and sadness, but after some tears his life returned to normal. During his third session with the psychologist, mere weeks after learning of Marcus's suicide, he found himself wondering, "Why am I still meeting with this lady?"

Sebastian: Recovery Group

After learning about the suicide, Sebastian seemed to really struggle. His mother was most concerned by his decreased appetite and frequent nightmares. When he returned to school, the teachers who remembered Sebastian all agreed that he was not himself. In the first several meetings with the school psychologist, Sebastian was able to process his feelings of anger, confusion, and sadness about the loss of his friend and shared that he could not understand why Marcus would kill himself. As the weeks passed, Sebastian still experienced some sadness related to the loss of his friend, but his nightmares started decreasing in frequency, and his appetite slowly returned. A couple of months into the new school year, his mother remarked that she felt like she had her son back.

Brian: Chronic Group

Brian was distraught when he heard about Marcus. He immediately started isolating himself from his family and friends. At home he spent long hours in his room, and at school he kept headphones in his ears whenever possible. He attended his meetings with the school psychologist but was very shut down in speaking with her, and they often spent the sessions in silence. Large, dark circles became a long-term feature of his face, and he told his parents that he just couldn't seem to fall asleep. His grades were lower than during the previous year, and his teachers remarked that he didn't seem to care about any of his classes.

Kenny, Sebastian, and Brian all went to the same school and were each part of the same group of friends, and yet they followed divergent paths in how they responded to the same traumatic event. Each one needed help in his own way.

Has My Child Been Traumatized?

How do you determine which group your child falls into? Like much of life, solving this question is often a question of timing.

When diagnosing patients after exposure to a potentially traumatic event, one of the first things I always consider is length of time from the exposure to the event. Symptoms that are normal and healthy in the days following an event could be seen as more troublesome a month out. A child who acts disturbed or scared immediately after an event can turn out to be healthy a short time later. It's important to keep in mind a time frame when considering a child's symptoms and trying to determine if the child has been traumatized.

In the immediate aftermath of a potentially traumatic event, your child may exhibit the following:

- Denial and disbelief
- Feelings of shock

- Emotional numbness

- Sense of powerlessness

- Somatic symptoms (headaches, stomachaches, etc.)

- Difficulty concentrating

- Nightmares

- Decrease or increase in appetite

- Difficulty falling or staying asleep or sleeping too much

- Jumpiness

- Increased negative feelings like fear, horror, anger, guilt

- Increased negative thoughts like "The world is not a safe place"

All of these symptoms—when experienced in mild degrees immediately following an adverse event—are perfectly normal. These are not a cause for concern. Children in the resilient class may experience a few of these symptoms to a benign degree, only to have them fade in the days and weeks after the event without professional support or intervention. A child in the recovery class may experience these symptoms with a greater frequency, intensity, and/or duration but will also recover. In their cases, some supportive interventions may be helpful. It is also worth noting that therapy interventions for children experiencing mild to moderate symptoms in the days and weeks following a trauma can look markedly different from the type of therapy a child with chronic symptoms would receive. For example, many trauma therapists use "watchful waiting"—monitoring kids for any symptoms—teach coping skills, and use supportive interventions for children who have just recently experienced an adverse event. On the other hand, for children who have ongoing symptoms that are interfering with their day-to-day life, a directive trauma protocol—a therapeutic intervention specifically developed to address trauma—is likely called for.

But beware the unintended impact an early, intense call for therapeutic support can have. In fact, an overreaction from parents can be one of the bigger dangers for resilient children.

A message to all the well-meaning, cautious caregivers: While it can feel empowering to try to get your child connected to professional psychological services immediately, you can risk inadvertently worsening your child's symptoms in the process. Children's thoughts and feelings about scary events are impacted by the reactions of adults around them. This is called *social referencing,* a concept originally studied in the 1980s by Mary Klinnert and her colleagues, and it's something that naturally wanes as children grow up. The point is this: Adults calling attention to the traumatic nature of an event may actually worsen posttraumatic stress symptoms in some children. Whether consciously or unconsciously, kids look up to adults. If you act like an event was scary or dangerous, then kids will treat it that way. Make sure to look to your child for guidance. If your kid doesn't seem worried, then you shouldn't worry either.

Think about it this way: A cousin your child met a few times was killed in a sudden, gruesome manner. You notice your own posttraumatic stress symptoms and are convinced that after hearing about this sudden death your entire family will be traumatized. But to your kid, this relative is someone she barely knows and has little to no emotional connection with, and this isn't something that impacts her life in any way she can discern. After being scooted immediately into therapy or pressured repeatedly to talk about her feelings surrounding this loss, she may come to think, "Oh wow, this is actually a big scary deal," rather than "I think I remember him from Thanksgiving last year—was he the one with the loud laugh?"

But what if these symptoms last for more than just a few days or weeks? Or what if they seem more intense than mild? If your child seems to be struggling with chronic symptoms or is experiencing symptoms that interfere with his life at home, at school, or with friends, it might be time to seek professional help.

Other times, parents might think a scary experience was "no big deal" and feel puzzled by stress symptoms popping up in their children. Consider this example: You are walking the dog with your six-year-old daughter one cold winter evening. You slip on the ice, hitting your head, and lose consciousness for a minute. Your neighbor, a doctor, comes out to help and stays with your daughter while you get checked out at a local urgent care. It turns out you have a mild concussion, but you're able to get home in time to put your daughter to bed. You call it a funny story and move on, but your daughter starts acting in strange ways, like desperately pleading with you not to walk the dog.

One of the first things a therapist may do is evaluate your child's symptoms to see if they meet criteria for PTSD or any of the other common trauma- and stressor-related disorders. It might be helpful for you to have an overview of what these disorders are to see if any of them resonate with you.

Trauma- and Stressor-Related Disorders

If you are one of the many parents who turned to Dr. Google for a free consultation after your child's exposure to a scary event, you may have come across terms like *posttraumatic stress, acute stress reaction, reactive attachment disorder*, or many of the other trauma- and stressor-related disorders that mental health professionals sometimes diagnose. The importance of diagnoses is that they can often help guide therapeutic treatment and inform therapists about which interventions might be most effective for your child. Mental health professionals assign these diagnoses only after careful examination—Dr. Google isn't enough. But understanding these terms can help you see the full spectrum of how mental health professionals understand and think about trauma. While there is nuance, each diagnosis comes with its own best practices for understanding where trauma came from and how it can best be treated.

Posttraumatic Stress Disorder

PTSD is a psychiatric disorder that can develop after someone has experienced a potentially traumatic event. In mainstream culture, the pervasive belief is that this is a diagnosis typically reserved for soldiers and veterans. While trauma diagnoses were first developed to help serve this population, people of any age who have experienced or witnessed any one of the events described above can also meet criteria for PTSD.

To meet criteria for PTSD, that is, to be diagnosed by a mental health professional, your older child or adolescent must have experienced the following:

- Had direct exposure to the adverse experience (as a passenger in a horrifying car accident, for example)
- Witnessed the experience (for instance, observed the horrifying crash happen right in front of him)
- Learned that a relative or close friend was exposed to the experience (such as learning a relative is in critical condition after a car accident)

or

- Had indirect exposure to aversive details of the trauma (for example, doing a police officer ride-along and responding to the crash)

Very young children (six and under) also must have had direct exposure, witnessed the experience, or learned about it happening to a close friend or relative, but a bigger emphasis is placed on incidents involving primary caregivers. As in the example on page 34, a young child isn't likely to be fazed if a relative she met only a few times is killed in a freak accident, but if the child's primary caregiver who helps get the child up every morning, fixes breakfast, and greets the child upon the child's return home from school has to stay in the hospital for a week following a serious accident, this would be scarier to little ones.

In addition to exposure to an adverse event, your child would also have symptoms in the following clusters:

- Intrusive symptoms, such as recurrent nightmares, flashbacks, or repeated intrusive thoughts about the trauma. For very young children (six and under), this could appear in their play (such as reenacting the adverse event over and over again).

- Avoidance symptoms, including attempts to avoid people, places, and things that may remind your child of the scary experience or refusal to talk about or remember important parts of the event.

- Arousal symptoms, including being jumpy or easily startled, experiencing difficulty with concentration and/or sleep, and irritability.

- Changes in thoughts and feelings, including having new negative thoughts about herself or the world, or experiencing new frequent feelings of fear, horror, anger, shame, or guilt.

Often these symptoms interfere with a child's ability to function in school, at home, and in relationships, which is also taken into account when making a diagnosis.

Do these symptoms sound familiar to you? If so, and it's been more than a month since your child was exposed to an adverse experience, your child might be experiencing PTSD. Or perhaps some of these symptoms resonate, but others sound less familiar.

Acute Stress Disorder

Another trauma- and stressor-related disorder is acute stress disorder (ASD), which has a lot of overlap with symptoms of PTSD but is diagnosed in days and weeks following exposure to the traumatic event, in contrast with PTSD, which is diagnosed with more long-standing symptoms that last more than one month. Another key difference between PTSD and ASD is that ASD is more likely to include symptoms of dissociation, such as not knowing where you are or feeling like you are outside of your body. Rates of ASD in trauma-exposed populations vary widely from 6 to 33 percent. According to the National Center for PTSD, rates of ASD differ based on the type of potentially traumatic event. Specifically, survivors of interpersonal violence show higher rates of ASD than survivors of accidents or natural disasters.

Adjustment Disorders

Adjustment disorders can also share some overlap with PTSD, but they do not require the presence of an adverse event. Sometimes more routine but still stressful events in life can cause stress symptoms in children. Consider any sort of major transition or adjustment, including moving to another state, the birth of a new sibling, or the death of an elderly grandparent due to a long-standing illness.

Reactive Attachment Disorder

Reactive attachment disorder (RAD) is a serious diagnosis that develops after long-standing trauma, typically abuse or neglect. Children who have been diagnosed with RAD have generally been exposed to such extensive trauma, starting at a very young age. They have learned attachment relationships are not safe. As a result, these kids might reject the comfort they could get from caregivers in times of distress. This is a rarer diagnosis and one that is typically seen in adopted children with extensive early trauma histories at the hands of their biological parents or in an orphanage.

Unclassified or Unspecified Trauma Disorder

Sometimes a child experiences symptoms of trauma but does not neatly fit into any of the diagnostic boxes described above. In these cases, if the symptoms have been going on for a while and seem to interfere with the child's life, a diagnosis of unclassified or unspecified trauma disorder may be appropriate.

When to Seek Professional Help

To provide some extra structure and guidance, if your child meets *any* one of the following criteria in group A after experiencing an adverse event, while simultaneously meeting a criterion in group B, it would be a safe bet to seek professional support. If your child does not have any of the following symptoms, it is still advised to seek professional help if your child requests it, or if you notice any other significant changes in your child's behavior.

Group A

❑ Lingering symptoms of hyperarousal (jumpiness, difficulty with concentration, irritability, changes in appetite or sleep habits)

❑ Lingering symptoms of avoidance (trying to stay away from people, places, things, and situations that might remind the child of the event)

❑ Lingering reexperiencing symptoms (nightmares, flashbacks of the event, unwanted upsetting memories or pictures related to the event that pop up in the child's mind, dissociation symptoms such as the child feeling like they are outside of their body)

❑ Lingering negative thoughts or feelings about the world,

herself, or others (feelings of sadness, fear, anger, guilt, or shame, or thoughts like "I will never be okay again" or "the world is a completely dangerous place")

Group B

❑ These symptoms seem to interfere with home life (increased fights with siblings and/or parents, increased isolation and avoidance of family activities)

❑ These symptoms seem to interfere with social life (increased fights with friends, decreased interest in socializing, decreased social outings)

❑ These symptoms seem to interfere with school life (increased teacher reports of acting out in class, inattention in class, increased skipping class, falling grades)

❑ These symptoms interfere with their ability to take care of themselves in tasks of daily life (eating, sleeping, bathing)

The reason that I include the last four check boxes is that some people may have some minimal stress symptoms throughout their lives that are no cause for concern. Take for example the startle response. Imagine you're at work, in a quiet office, when all of a sudden you hear a loud crash. Do you and your coworkers flinch? While your coworker to the left might have barely noticed, staying focused on his current task, maybe the colleague on your right looks like a frightened kitten, hair on the back of her arm standing at attention, pupils constricted. Perhaps you flinched a bit, felt unsettled, but easily zeroed back in on your work after seeing it was a stack of binders that fell over. None of these responses alone, even your coworker's exaggerated startle response, is indicative of trauma. Many people go through their lives with at least one or two symptoms that align with posttraumatic stress, but it doesn't mean they are traumatized. If, however, you or a coworker were so startled by a sudden loud noise that you were unable to focus on your work for the rest of the day, that might indicate this is an issue you need to take seriously.

While mental health professionals rely on different specific diagnoses to help them categorize and treat people dealing with trauma, it really does all come down to this key question: *Is someone exhibiting symptoms, and are those symptoms interfering with everyday life?* If you can answer that question about your child, then you have taken the first critical step to understanding what your child needs to heal, which may be professional help in addition to your skillful, supportive parenting.

Differences across Ages

Different kids may exhibit similar symptoms or follow similar trajectories, but it is important to keep in mind that age remains another key dividing line in what you should look for. Trauma symptoms vary widely across age ranges. Very young children tend to be clingier and more fearful. Adolescents tend to respond by withdrawing and engaging in more risk-taking, impulsive behavior. Here are some more specifics about different symptoms across the developmental ages:

Infants and Young Toddlers

For children from birth to around age two, trauma symptoms include increased or new separation anxiety that consists of the fear of being separated from their primary caregiver *or* a fear of strangers even when their primary caregiver is close, increased fussiness and crying around sleep and mealtimes, and increased clinginess, even if you are home alone with your child.

Consider this example: Charlie, eighteen months old, was suddenly separated from his mother for a month after she flew out of state to care for her own ailing mother in home hospice. Charlie was adequately cared for by his father and paternal grandparents, never missing a meal or cuddle, but he had not spent a lot of time with his paternal grandparents prior to this month, and the seemingly easygoing tyke would cry and scream until he was hoarse when his father left for work in the mornings.

Children Ages Two through Six

For this age group, trauma symptoms include increased tearfulness, increased clinginess, avoiding nap time and bedtime (refusing to stay in their bedroom at night, attempts to sneak into parents' bedroom, tantrumming to avoid bedtime), increased irritability, and behavioral regression (wetting the bed long after successful toilet training, thumb sucking, talking "like a baby").

Consider this example: Dev, five, had been looking forward to swim lessons for weeks. He had had a wonderful experience last season but was dismayed to learn his old teacher wasn't returning. Instead, Dev was paired with a first-time teacher, and during their first session, when he told Dev he had his hands right underneath him, he slipped under the water and thrashed about for 10 seconds before the instructor scooped him up. Dev immediately threw up all over himself. His mother, who was watching the lesson, ran over and told the teacher they were done for the day. She later promised Dev they would not be seeing that teacher again. She thought these assurances would be enough to comfort Dev, but, months after this incident, his parents find he still sneaks into their room every night and sleeps on the floor, refusing to sleep in his own room by himself. Any attempt at redirecting him back to his own room is met with a massive tantrum.

Children Ages Seven through Twelve

For these older kids, trauma symptoms include somatic symptoms (headaches, stomachaches), changes in sleep habits (sleeping more than usual, or less than usual, attempts to avoid sleep, nightmares), avoidance of peers and/or family, increased clinginess, increased irritability and/or aggression, increased jumpiness in response to sudden or loud noises, changes in eating behaviors (either eating significantly more or less than usual).

Becca, nine, was bullied and beaten up by two older children at school. The bullying took place over three months and escalated to one of the bullies pushing Becca off bleachers, breaking her arm in the process. The bullies were immediately expelled from school, but every morning during breakfast Becca starts complaining of intense stomachaches and says she can't go to school.

Adolescents

For teenagers, trauma symptoms include somatic symptoms (headaches, stomachaches), self-harming behaviors (cutting), substance abuse, other impulsive behaviors (driving too fast, not wearing a seat belt), changes in sleep (too much or too little), changes in eating (too much or too little, sometimes with accompanying weight gain or weight loss), and difficulty with concentration, especially in school.

Consider this example: Jani, seventeen, was sexually assaulted by a classmate at a party one weekend. Jani's friends were able to interrupt part of the assault, but she was still pretty shaken up by it. Since the party, Jani tells her friends that she is "totally fine," but they notice some big changes. A couple weeks after the party, they notice Jani carrying a water bottle filled with vodka to school and are shocked when their normally cautious friend tries to drive home while clearly drunk.

As kids grow older, they become more mature and complex individuals, and their trauma symptoms change along with them. It will be more difficult to ascertain what a teenager is going through than a preschooler. Routine teenage behavior can sometimes look like a trauma response—impulsive decision making stands out as both a hallmark of adolescence and a symptom of trauma. Remember to be patient with your teen. There are specific tactics for interacting with teenagers who may have suffered from trauma that we'll discuss in depth in Chapter 10.

All of this can feel overwhelming. Considering symptomatology, time frame, and age range can be a lot for a parent to keep in mind. Don't worry. If I had to identify one take-home message, it would be this: If your child's symptoms seem to be lingering and interfere with the child's everyday life, it's time to call in a professional. If your child seems to be struggling before you can determine if his symptoms are lingering, or you feel like you just don't know if he could benefit from therapy, a consult with a therapist is a good idea and likely will not hurt anyone. Just beware the potential pitfalls of trying to force your child into regular therapy if she is resistant or is insisting everything is okay. If your child is resistant to therapy but you are still worried, this would be the time for you to schedule a therapeutic consultation for yourself. Your own therapist can support and guide you in when and how to take action so that you can best help your child.

Kids of every age can be resilient. In my clinical experience, a strong parent–child relationship is the factor most predictive of resilience and healing. The simple fact that you're reading this book means that you care about your child and want to help—and you're already on the path to success. The next chapter will delve further into the parent–child relationship and give you concrete, easy-to-use tools to enhance your relationship with your child and facilitate healing.

3

You Are the Key to Helping Your Child Heal

If you read Chapters 1 and 2, you probably have a fairly clear idea of whether your child has suffered trauma from exposure to an adverse experience. You should also have some understanding of which risk and protective factors have contributed to how your child is feeling right now. A lot might be at work in your child's mind, and it's not always easy to sort out. But there is one core lesson in all this: a strong parent–child relationship is one of the most robust components in helping a child heal from trauma. This isn't just my own observation as a psychologist—it is backed by academic research. Building an even stronger relationship with your child in the aftermath of a potentially traumatic event will not only lay the foundation for healing but can also buffer your child from some of the ill effects of future traumas.

I want to acknowledge right up front, however, that building this relationship isn't always easy. Parents can be busy with work and other family obligations. Kids can be overwhelmed with school and extra-curricular activities. So many things in life can get in the way. That's why, after reviewing exactly how a close parent–child relationship can help a child heal, this chapter offers concrete, easy-to-implement relationship-building skills, including quality time, mentalizing, praise, active listening, and enjoyment. All of these skills will benefit any parent–child relationship but are essential to facilitating the healing process for a traumatized child.

The Importance of Attachment

One spring morning my husband decided to take our then eighteen-month-old daughter for a ride in a new red wagon she had just received as a gift. He was pulling her behind him, running across the yard in his old shoes with worn-out treads, and he slipped and fell. The wagon tipped over, and our toddler careened out of her ride and onto the grass, bumping her head. She cried out for Mama. I ran to her. But instead of reaching out to me for a kiss or hug, she urgently pointed to the grass, dropped to all fours, gently tapped her head against the ground, and gazed back at me. My preverbal sweetheart was trying to show me exactly what had happened. She did this a few more times, deeply wanting me to understand her scary experience. After I gave her some comfort and verbalized her experience, she settled down and let out a big sigh.

Jon Allen, a psychologist and mentor of mine, once shared this straightforward summary of what we know about coping: "The single best way we know to deal with emotional pain is to connect to others to whom we feel securely attached." For children, the most powerful attachment relationship is often with a primary caregiver—that means you. As a primary caregiver, you are uniquely positioned to help your child heal from a traumatic experience. You don't have to be exceptionally empathic or have any special skills as a therapist. You just have to foster a secure attachment relationship between yourself and your child.

Attachment and Trauma

At its core, attachment is the emotional bond we share with another person. While this chapter will focus on the importance of the attachment bond between parent and child, it is important to note that we all have many attachments in our lives—to our spouses, close friends, even colleagues. We never outgrow the need for attachment relationships; whenever we are in a painful place, the best medicine we have is connection to these relationships.

One study that illustrates the power of the attachment relationship measured how simply having your hand held by an attachment figure could help protect your brain against distress. In 2006, neuroscientist James Coan and his colleagues identified happily married couples, brought them into his lab, and, after a visit in which the couples were fully informed that the experiment would include minor electric shocks, proceeded to deliver mild electric shocks to the wife. The wives were assigned to one of three experimental conditions: in one group the wives were allowed to hold their husbands' hands throughout the shocks; the wives in another group could hold the hand of an anonymous male experimenter; and the wives in the third group were not offered any hand to hold. The results were straightforward: As you might have guessed, the women holding their husbands' hands fared the best, and their brains showed the least threat-activated response to impending shocks. The women without a hand to hold had the highest neural threat response. But it wasn't just about holding hands. Among the women paired with their spouses, the experimenters found that couples with higher reported marital relationship satisfaction had even less of a stress response than their slightly less satisfied peers. The bottom line: receiving comfort from and connection to our primary attachment figures bolsters our ability to tolerate distress.

When it comes to traumatized children, they are undoubtedly experiencing more distress than a woman who participated in a study knowing she would be receiving electric shocks. More than ever, they need an available, reliable hand to hold. As reviewed in Chapter 1, after a potentially traumatic experience your child's understanding of herself and the world around her may be rocked. By standing with her and being available to her—extending your hand, so to speak—you are telling your child she is not alone in this confusing and scary time. She has a grounded, trusted figure to understand her, keep her safe, and see her through.

Specifically, secure attachment can help counter your child's trauma symptoms in these ways:

- Your child will not be alone in his distress, making the distress easier to manage.

- Your child will gain understanding and acceptance instead of being isolated and feeling shame.

- You can serve as a trusted authority figure who can help guide healing, lending support and inspiring hope.

- You can erect boundaries to help keep your child safe, preventing future traumatization and creating a sense of felt safety.

But how do you get to that point where your child will reach out and take your outstretched hand? As I mentioned in Chapter 2, if you cared enough to buy a book about parenting a traumatized child, you are likely well on your way! Think back to when your child was an infant. If he cried, would you (or another primary caregiver) reliably go to his aid? Offer him a clean diaper, some milk, or just some good old-fashioned soothing? If so, wonderful. This is how a secure attachment relationship develops. Over days, weeks, and months of your responding in his cries for help, he has learned that he has someone who will reliably and consistently be available to him. Before his first birthday, he will have developed confidence in his relationship with his primary caregivers and will be more likely to reach out to them in his time of need.

Unfortunately, not every infant has the experience of a reliable caregiver. This can be due to a variety of different factors. Sometimes parents of newborns are overwhelmed by a needy older sibling, a demanding work schedule, or simply the stress of adjusting to life as a new parent. In this circumstance, an infant may sense that their needs will be met only if they make a giant fuss, getting purple in the face and shrieking at a high decibel level. This type of attachment style could be labeled as *insecure*. This baby might be anxious or ambivalent about reaching out in response to their needs. Alternatively, a baby could also get the sense that caregivers get overwhelmed by their cries. Perhaps Mother suffers from perinatal depression or Father is terrified by all of his new responsibilities, checking out emotionally whenever the baby expresses distress. In a worst-case scenario, one parent might even become abusive to their child in response to the baby's cries. These babies may develop a different type of insecure attachment style, electing to "go it alone" rather than turn toward Mom or Dad after a scary experience. See the box on the next page for those cases in which trauma stems from abuse at the hands of one parent.

Relationship-Building Skills

So what to do if your child was never securely attached? Or if everything seemed to be going well in childhood, but you sense your teen is drifting away in early adolescence? Or perhaps you thought your child was securely attached prior to the potentially traumatic event but feel she is pushing you away now? Even though attachment styles do not change easily, through a variety of relationship-building skills you can foster a more secure attachment with your child, so she will feel empowered to reach her little hand out and meet you halfway when struggling with the distressing and painful thoughts and feelings that sometimes accompany an adverse experience.

Quality Time

The first relationship-enhancing skill I always prescribe to parents of traumatized children is quality time.

Parents might not understand how they provide a sense of safety for their kids. For example, I have worked with many kids who suddenly develop a fear of the dark after a trauma, even if the original

When Trauma Involves an Attachment Figure

Trauma involving primary caregivers is less rare than you would think. Whether Mom is injured in a car crash, Dad suddenly gets diagnosed with an aggressive cancer, or one parent is abusive to another family member, these types of potentially traumatic experiences can sting the most. Especially in the youngest children, who are most dependent on their caregivers, the loss or threat of loss of a primary caregiver can be a huge disturbance to their attachment system. The good news? Research into attachment has consistently demonstrated that it takes only one secure attachment to a primary caregiver for a child to develop into a healthy, high-functioning adult. This attachment figure need not be Mom or Dad, but could be any biological relative, foster or adoptive parent, or a surrogate caregiver. As long as you are consistently available and reliable, your little one has all he needs.

event was not related to the nighttime or darkness. The child will cope with that fear by barging into the parents' room in the middle of the night and asking to join them in bed or by insisting that a parent come back to sleep in the child's room. The real fear in these situations isn't the lack of light, but of being *alone* in the dark without the calming presence of a parent. The dark isn't so scary when Mom or Dad is there to snuggle.

No matter what the traumatic experience may have been, a child will probably feel overwhelmed, anxious, saddened, or stressed after a scary event. Intimate, quality time with you—whether it is a snuggle in bed or a quick walk around the block—can help alleviate some of the pangs of trauma. Of course, parents cannot provide quality time to their child 24/7—that's not the goal. Instead, incorporating quality time as part of the daily routine helps children internalize the sense that Mom or Dad is with them when they need it the most. Parents don't need to be there physically if kids can feel it emotionally. The challenge is in getting kids to that point.

What Is Quality Time?

Quality time can be almost anything.

Literally anything.

It can be doing a puzzle, watching sports, or in the case of my patient from the Introduction, playing mini-golf. The critical aspect of quality time isn't the activity—it's that the practice involves giving undivided attention to a single person. In the context of the family system, quality time can be spent between spouses, siblings, or parent and child. What sets quality time apart from other one-on-one time is that the parent and child should be connecting with each other in a way that is meaningful. The literature agrees: Research into parenting practices consistently shows that the quality of time, rather than the quantity, has the greatest impact on child development. Even watching television with your child can be quality time if you're both engaged with the show on the screen together—laughing at the same funny bits, speculating about what's going to happen next, and the like. If your child is watching but you're absorbed by your iPhone, your child naturally won't feel your presence or the shared experience.

The single greatest benefit of quality time is the deepening of the parent–child relationship, creating a strong attachment bond. In addition to promoting healing from an adverse event, a strong attachment bond between parent and child has numerous psychosocial benefits, including:

- Increased self-esteem
- Decreased vulnerability to child sexual abuse
- Decreased or delayed use of drugs and alcohol
- Improved academic achievement
- Improved social skills

As you will read in Chapters 4–10, children who have been exposed to adverse events may end up struggling with problems related to friendships, family relationships, schoolwork, and general well-being. Bolstering your child with a strong, secure attachment relationship might provide the child with armor against some of these negative effects.

A close attachment bond not only has benefits for psychosocial outcomes but also affects physical health later in life. Research has found that children who experience secure attachments to caregivers, warm parenting, and decreased parental conflict exhibit less secretion of stress hormones. As reviewed in Chapter 1, long-term activation of the body's stress hormones is associated with a number of poor outcomes, including social outcomes like struggling to complete schooling, an increased risk of crime and violence involvement, and increased use of alcohol and drugs, and health outcomes like greater susceptibility to heart disease, mental health disorders, and early death. But it's not all doom and gloom: think of a strong parent–child relationship as a vaccine against some of the ill effects of trauma. While you might not be able to prevent all of the physical, psychological, and social outcomes after an adverse event, you can provide your child with a good deal of protection that lessens the impact. How wonderful that something as simple as quality time in childhood can help lay the foundation for a healthy life.

How Do You Make Time Together Quality Time?

So how do you actually have quality time with your child? The first step is to find an activity the child might feel excited about. On some days, when you both have a flexible schedule, quality time might look like a drive to the beach to play in the waves together. On other days, when you are both scrambling with work and school, it could be something as simple as walking the dog together. Take a few moments to consider some of the ideas below with your child or teen and try to identify a few activities that both of you might find engaging. Keep in mind that it does not matter what you and your child elect to do, so long as you are doing it together.

- Bake a cake
- Collaborate on a scrapbook
- Have side-by-side reading time
- Play a video game
- Go on a bike ride
- Garden
- Identify and collaborate on a home-improvement project of your child's choice
- Plan a future vacation
- Visit a botanical garden
- Practice yoga
- Play a board game
- Watch a movie
- Attend a sporting event
- Volunteer
- Go for a jog

Quality time is an intervention that may sound obvious, but many parents struggle to implement it. Perhaps this was easier when your child was very young, when your child was more agreeable, before

What about Toddlers?

It may seem like more trouble than it's worth to try to lug your toddler to a botanical garden or to involve them in a baking experiment. Very young children—even up to age six—are often just as thrilled by a few minutes of one-on-one child-directed play with you. Put on some comfortable clothes, get on the floor with them, and let them lead you wherever their creativity takes them.

the siblings came along, or before you started taking on more responsibility at work. Although it may be hard to acknowledge, many parents go through periods of time when they don't particularly like spending one-on-one time with their child. This is perfectly normal and natural. At the same time, it is all the more important to find a way to make this time successful and enjoyable for you both.

I once worked with a single mother, Amy, who had two children in elementary school. The entire family was traumatized after her husband was arrested and convicted for sexual assault. Amy was a bright and capable woman who was doing her best to keep her family sane. While she had been a stay-at-home mother, her husband's incarceration meant she had to find a job after being out of work for a decade, all while balancing the everyday mental and physical load of single parenthood. This poor mom was completely drained. Whenever her kids would act out, whether getting into physical fights with each other or being disrespectful to her, she could feel the anger and resentment bubbling up inside of her. All she wanted, desperately, was some time alone—something that she no doubt needed! That's why, when I spoke to Amy about quality time as an intervention, she looked at me

Beware of Overengagement

While we want parents to be engaged in their quality-time activity with their child, some parents may go too far and overwhelm their child. Picture a fed-up teenager constantly fielding questions from her mother about the plot of a new television show they are watching together. For parents tending toward overengagement, it might be helpful to envision yourself sitting on your hands. Use that imagery to try to refrain from peppering your child with too much personal involvement during quality time. Spending time together should feel like a nice hug, not a squeeze from a boa constrictor.

like I was instead suggesting she go for a swim with two particularly hungry great white sharks. However, after we looked at her schedule together, we found small ways she could spend time alone with each child, and she agreed to give it a try. Amy took up baking with her daughter, and they both quickly came to look forward to trying new recipes. The time immediately after school was reserved for her son— he and Amy would take their miniature poodle to the dog park, just the two of them. Weeks later she described feeling surprised by how much she enjoyed the quality time and how she noticed a decrease in the physical fights, parental disrespect, and other trauma symptoms since implementing the practice. With her family feeling more settled after enduring a traumatic experience, Amy even found more opportunities for some well-deserved time to herself.

Mentalizing

Mentalizing is a fancy-sounding term for a simple concept that can deepen your relationship with your child. It refers to the process by which we think about and make sense of other people's mental states, as well as our own. It harks back to Descartes's "I think, therefore I am," and was even developed into its own therapeutic treatment by Drs. Anthony Bateman and Peter Fonagy (see more about mentalization-based treatment in Chapter 11). Overall, it's about being curious about what's going on in someone else's mind, as well as your own. For the purposes of this book, think of it as imagining what it might be like to be in your child's shoes, or a sort of cognitive practice of empathy. To understand your child's inner experience, let curiosity, respect, and compassion lead the way.

Many of us do this already, only to be waylaid when we encounter our own strong emotions or uncomfortable thoughts. Our child does something that frustrates us to no end, and it gets pretty hard to stay curious about *why* he might have done this thing that frustrated us. Feeling this type of frustration—or any other strong negative emotion—shuts down our ability to mentalize. It's hard to be curious and think about another person's experience when we are stuck in our own experience.

The tricky thing about this is that the confusing, frustrating, infuriating behaviors of traumatized children frequently stem from their emotional distress. These are the moments they need their primary attachment figure the most—but at the same time, these are often moments when parents want to shut down or reprimand their child, rather than try to understand the child.

Yasmin, a junior at her local high school, is the star of her school's soccer team. Her parents have spent lots of time and money carting her to practices and games and making sure she has the best equipment, despite some financial struggles. The entire family is thrilled when they hear a college scout will be attending an end-of-season game and are initially shocked and furious when Yasmin doesn't show up. They learn from another parent in the stands that Yasmin's boyfriend had broken up with her just before the big game.

A nonmentalizing approach: After getting home, Yasmin's parents tear into her about how selfish and stupid she was for missing her shot with the college scout. They lecture her about how much they have sacrificed so that she could have this opportunity and how her future will be worse because of her shortsighted decision to skip the game. Yasmin refuses to make eye contact with her parents during this lecture, but they can see the tears rolling down her cheeks. She spends the next day locked in her room, refusing to eat or talk to anyone.

A mentalizing approach: After getting home, Yasmin's parents share what they have heard about the breakup and gently inquire if that's why she missed the game. Their tone is one of curiosity, rather than blame and anger, and they can imagine their daughter is feeling rejected and sad. Instead of feeling shut down, belittled, and blamed by her parents, Yasmin feels supported. She shares that actually she has been trying to break up with her boyfriend for months, but he has threatened to send a nude photo of her to the entire school if she does not stay with him. Though she has relented and stayed with him, the day of her big game he shared the photo with his friends. She says that she felt humiliated and ashamed and didn't know what to do. She also shares her worries that his friends would harass her from the stands and her belief that there was no way she could keep her head in the game with all of this stress, and she did not want to embarrass herself in front of the college scout. Yasmin and her parents spend that evening coming up with a plan for how to respond to his exploitation.

As demonstrated in Yasmin's story, when you mentalize your children, they are more likely to feel comfortable opening up to you, deepening your attachment relationship. It didn't matter that Yasmin's parents were initially wrong about what was going on in her mind; when they approached her with curiosity and compassion, she felt supported enough to share her true experience with them.

When your child does something that frustrates or confuses you, if you can approach him with the same curiosity and compassion rather than anger and blame, you will be sending the message that you want to understand him rather than punish him, making him more likely to open up and feel close to you. In addition to deepening the relationship, if your child is open with you about a potentially traumatic experience, you can help. In the vignette above, Yasmin likely didn't consider any type of recourse over the months that this boy was exploiting her. Now that her parents are in the loop, they can help her take action to protect herself and prevent further traumatization.

Praise

Praise is a wonderful relationship-enhancing skill for a number of different reasons. First, praising a child properly for a specific behavior makes that behavior more likely to occur again. When you regularly praise your child for behaviors you like to see, they are more likely to become part of your child's behavioral repertoire. When your child is behaving in ways that are pleasing to you, you will enjoy your time together a lot more, and your child will pick up on that too.

So what does proper praise look like?

Picture your daughter playing with her younger brother in the family room. You notice her sharing her prized magnetic tiles with him. This would be a perfect opportunity to heap praise on your daughter. While a "Good girl!" would certainly be appreciated, the more specific and concrete you can be with your praise, the better. With this example, ideal praise might be "I love how you shared your tiles with your brother!" As your daughter continues to get this positive reinforcement from you, she will be more likely to share with her brother—especially in front of you, which will hopefully engender feelings of pride and closeness in both of you.

Praise is also a good relationship-deepening practice because it helps children feel good about themselves and creates the sense that they will feel good about themselves in the context of their relationship with you. Regular, specific praise tells them that they are doing a good job at home and that the people they depend on most approve of them.

Praise is included as an intervention in this chapter because of how it enhances the parent–child relationship. At the same time, after exposure to a potentially traumatic event, children's sense of themselves and the world can be shattered. Instead of feeling like their regular, competent selves, they may have suffered a drop in their self-esteem. Getting the consistent message that they're doing a good job on their specific tasks at home can go a long way in grounding them and helping them to feel good about themselves.

Active Listening

Active listening is one of the first skills in a new therapist's playbook. Active listening is important because it lets the person you're listening to know that you are truly engaging with her, that you're paying attention to what she is saying, that you are understanding her. When a patient describes to me a terrifying ordeal that felt scary and overwhelming, I might reply, "It sounds like you were feeling terrified." This would help my patient feel understood and know that I'm paying attention. It would also help the person feel more comfortable in continuing to share with me, thereby building our closeness.

While it would be great if you could regularly reflect your child's most vulnerable feelings back to them, children don't always share these types of emotions with parents. Active listening can also be practiced in less emotionally charged situations, while still having the same impact of enhancing the relationship. If your child shares with you that he wants to get his math homework done before walking the dog because he's feeling nervous about getting it done by a deadline, you could reflect this statement by saying, "I hear ya. That math work is stressing you out and you just want to get it off your plate."

For very young children, an ideal time to practice this new skill could be while you play together. If your little one describes taking her stuffed animals for a ride in the wagon, you might try something like "You're taking your bears and puppies for a ride around the room." This lets her know she is being understood and gives her a sense that Mom or Dad is paying attention.

A word of caution: Children of all ages can get annoyed if your reflections parrot them exactly. A helpful way to think about reflecting is trying to summarize or put what your child is saying in your own words. You're trying to let children know you hear them and you understand them, not trying to copy or mimic them, which would be annoying to any of us.

Another benefit of practicing active listening with your child is that the child will be able to let you know if you get it wrong. If you mishear or misinterpret something your child is saying and reflect back something the child didn't mean, he can then let you know that, helping you understand better.

Overall, active listening is a wonderful relationship-building skill because it helps children feel heard and paid attention to. This gives them the sense that they matter to you and that you are available for them. Though you'll likely be practicing active listening most in response to neutral stimuli like play time or math homework, they will develop the sense that their primary caregiver is both responsive and available, fostering that secure attachment that is invaluable to the traumatized child.

Additionally, a child who does want to open up to you about trauma-related thoughts or feelings will become more comfortable and less ambivalent about doing so with the general sense that in conversation you do a good job of listening to and understanding them.

Enjoyment

Contrary to what social media might lead some to believe, not every part of parenting is fun or enjoyable. From the sleepless newborn nights to toddler toilet training, from navigating the awkward beginnings of puberty in early adolescence to teenage power struggles, a lot of blood, sweat, and tears is involved in raising another human being. At the same time, there is a lot to love and relish. The key thing with enjoyment is letting your children see you loving to spend time with them. Instead of just savoring those moments after all your children are bathed and in bed and you finally have a couple minutes to yourself, try to show your enjoyment as you feel it throughout the day.

This practice most easily ties back to quality time—finding something that you both enjoy doing and doing it together. While doing it, verbalize your enjoyment. A simple "I love baking cookies with you" will go a long way (if it is sincere). Another way to demonstrate this could be if your family has a practice of sharing the highs and lows of the day around the dinner table. Make sure every now and then to identify the highlight of your day as something you did with your child.

Showing your enjoyment of your children communicates that you like them and that they in turn are likable. This will do wonders for both their self-esteem and your parent–child relationship.

Additionally, traumatized children are more likely to believe there is something wrong with them or they are deficient in some way. This harks back to our discussion of schemas in Chapter 1. If your child harbored the commonly held belief that "good things happen to good people, and bad things happen to bad people," experiencing a "bad" or distressing event might send the child the inaccurate message that she is a bad person. By demonstrating that your child is enjoyable (and worthy of your time, your understanding, and your praise), you will help buoy your child's self-esteem, setting her on the path of healing.

The *Don'ts* of Creating a Secure Attachment

While quality time, mentalizing, praise, reflections, and enjoyment will all help foster a secure attachment relationship with your child, there are several communication practices that can shut down the development of a good bond in its tracks.

Commands without Rationale

No one likes being told what to do. Whether toddler, teen, or adult, many of us bristle at direct commands, even if we wouldn't necessarily mind the task we are being commanded to do. Of course, sometimes our kids *do* need directives—they need to wear their seat belt in the car, for example—but that doesn't undo the fact that commands are unpleasant to receive. They can feel controlling and inspire resistance. One way to make them more tolerable? Pair every request with a rationale. "We wear our seat belts to keep ourselves safe in the car." Providing a reason appeals to your child's sense of logic and demonstrates that you respect him. Every parent remembers the "Why?" stage in toddlerhood. Whether you're parenting a toddler or a teen, indulge your child! Connect every directive with a reason.

And please, take "because I said so" out of your vocabulary. This does not count as a rationale.

If you can't think of a good reason for giving the command, that's probably a good indicator you don't need to be giving it.

A constant barrage of demands communicates to your child that you don't trust her to take care of herself or function in your family. This can be harmful to a traumatized child's already vulnerable self-esteem and push her further away from you. By cutting down on commands and issuing only directives that have good reasons behind them, you're giving your child more freedom and demonstrating that you trust her and value her buy-in.

Sarcasm

While the content of sarcasm might sound similar to praise (for example, "Nice one, genius!" after your child makes a silly error), the intent behind sarcasm is to mock or express your displeasure. Depending on how it's communicated, it's typically either aggressive or passive aggressive, and it doesn't feel good. Fittingly, one of the origins of the word *sarcasm* comes from the Greek *sarkazein*, meaning to "tear flesh."

In addition to making your child feel bad, it might devalue authentic praise you give your child, especially in younger children, because your words are so similar.

You may find sarcasm funny, but the bottom line is that it's not nice, and a child in a vulnerable position doesn't need any extra hits, especially from the one (or more) people who are always supposed to be on their side.

Judging and Criticizing Your Child (Rather Than Focusing on Their Behaviors)

While everyone needs some feedback from time to time, it might be helpful to think of providing constructive feedback or guidance about children's behavior instead of critiquing them as people. When you're critical of your child, the child can internalize that something about him is bad or defective. If you instead focus on your child's behavior, it's easier for the child to take that less personally.

Picture this: Your son leaves a plate of pizza in his room, and you walk in and find it covered in flies. That behavior? Leaving pizza uncovered for days? Gross. Surely in need of some feedback. But your son himself? Who knows why he left the pizza. This one action does not make him a gross person.

Much like the other *don'ts*, this could be another hit to a wobbly sense of self or fragile self-esteem following a potentially traumatic event.

Each of these *don'ts* creates distance, resentment, and distrust in the parent–child relationship and can undermine self-esteem. Aim to stay away from these as much as possible. If you notice yourself having a hard time breaking the sarcasm habit or refraining from "because I said so!" this might be an indication that you could benefit from therapy of your own.

These "don't" behaviors don't just appear in a vacuum. You likely learned them from somewhere, and they can be hard to unlearn.

To wrap it up . . .

Being a kid can sometimes feel like being an explorer on the high seas. Much of the world is a mystery, and you have little direct knowledge about what awaits you over the horizon. Every day brings new wonders. When the sky is bright and you have the wind in your sails, life can be an exhilarating joy. But when dark clouds start to gather and the seas turn rocky, suddenly the world becomes a terrifying place—here be monsters. That's when your little explorer heads for safe harbor—that's you. Parents serve as a child's safe and secure base, where they can feel protected amid almost any type of tempest. And it's all the more important for children to know you're there for them after they've survived one of life's storms. Building a secure attachment relationship—that is, one within which your child can feel confident that you will be both available and reliable in times of distress—is paramount to helping a child heal from trauma.

By using quality time, mentalizing, praise, active listening, and enjoyment, and staying away from sarcasm, commands without rationale, and personal criticism and judgment, you can help foster this type of relationship and help your child heal.

PART II

Knowing What to Expect

4

Understanding Changes
in Your Child's Behavior

Mark, a nine-year-old only child, was playing in his front yard when he was attacked by a large stray dog. Thankfully, a good Samaritan witnessed the attack, chased the dog off, and called an ambulance. Mark suffered some deep cuts and needed stitches, but his body showed incredible resilience. It wasn't too long before Mark's wounds healed, and he started looking very much like his former self again— at least on the outside. On the inside, however, things seemed different. Mark had always had a close, largely conflict-free relationship with his parents, but after the attack he started to avoid them. Whenever his mother or father reached out to spend time with him, Mark rebuffed them. If they attempted to schedule some family time, he would scream at them to leave him alone. On one occasion, when his father entered Mark's room without knocking, Mark threw a book at him. This infuriated Mark's father, who then yelled at Mark, calling him "disrespectful" and "screwed up." Mark screamed back that he was running away and started shoving some belongings into his backpack. His mother overheard the entire interaction and sobbed to herself, thinking "I'm losing my child."

Behavioral Changes
and Posttraumatic Stress

As briefly addressed in Chapter 3, traumatized children may express their distress through uncharacteristic behaviors. Whether your child responds more like Yasmin (see pages 56–57) and withdraws from her passions, or like Mark (above), and exhibits increased aggression, at the heart of the matter is the fact that most of these behavioral changes are actually coping mechanisms. In a bid to protect themselves from perceived threats or uncomfortable emotions, it can actually be (at least initially) healthy for children to get angry and make themselves seem scary, throw a tearful tantrum, pull back, or even regress behaviorally. These behavioral changes are not necessarily intentional or even conscious.

As a parent, it can be confusing, disheartening, or even frustrating to see your child act in these strange new ways. But rest assured, your child probably feels even more confused and scared than you. Take comfort in knowing that these responses are normal and that the skills and understanding you gather in this book will help you make sense of and ameliorate them.

Behavioral Changes You Might See
in Your Child

Children can undergo many different types of behavioral changes after a trauma. These changes will often occur in the days following a scary event, but sometimes they'll appear even weeks or months later. Before you jump in to try to "fix" these changes, it is important to have some sort of understanding about the common classes of changes that you may encounter as well as why they pop up in traumatized children.

Some changes can be sudden and intense and appear to be more of an immediate physiological response than anything. This might look like your son flinching when someone taps him on the shoulder or your daughter running away when she encounters something that reminds her of the trauma. We call these sudden physiological responses *being triggered*, and triggers will be covered below and in depth in Chapter 5. Other behavioral changes may be gradual, building slowly over time and appearing to be less physiologically based and more psychologically driven. These behaviors, including increased emotionality and behavioral regression, minor and major misbehavior, withdrawal and avoidance, and impulsive behaviors, will be addressed in depth in Chapters 6–10. Regardless of which behavior changes your child may be exhibiting, it's important to focus on understanding the cause of these behaviors—which is often some form of self-protection—before you think about responding to them.

Triggers

In psychology, triggers are stimuli that remind the body of a past threat. Though the term has a bit of a controversial slant at present—some use it as a jab to indicate someone is being overly sensitive—it is actually rooted in a physiological survival instinct. Understanding this unconscious process of triggering is key to helping your child feel safe and supported.

Here's the way I break it down for my patients: Imagine you are camping in the wilderness and you see a bear. Suddenly, your heart starts pounding. Your breathing quickens. There's a tingle in your hands, and maybe they start to feel cold and clammy. Your body is getting you ready to fight the bear, run from the bear, or freeze in hopes that the bear does not perceive you as a threat and leaves you alone. All of these physiological reactions are the work of our sympathetic nervous system firing up a stress response that has kept humans safe over thousands of years: the fight–flight–freeze response. Think about it: Where would humanity be if we didn't freak out when we saw a bear? We would be inside the bear's stomach, of course.

A trauma trigger is something that reminds you of the bear—even if you're in a safe situation. Weeks after your camping trip, you are relaxing in your backyard when suddenly, out of the corner of your eye, you spot something large, brown, and fuzzy. You don't live anywhere near the woods. It's virtually impossible that a bear would have made its way to your backyard. You know in your mind that it's not a bear. But that doesn't stop your body from responding to this familiar threat. Just like on your camping trip, your heart races and pounds, you feel jittery, and you start to sweat. Quickly you realize it was your preteen son trying on his Chewbacca costume for Halloween next month, but it still takes some time for your heart rate to slow down and for you to relax again. You've just been triggered.

This is something that happens automatically. It all starts in your amygdala, the part of your brain that experiences fear. Your amygdala sends a warning to your hypothalamus, which is responsible for discharging crucial stress hormones. Once these hormones are released, our autonomic nervous system wakes up and triggers our sympathetic response, releasing even more stress hormones that cause changes all over our bodies.

These changes include:

- Faster breathing with more intense inhalations that increase alertness
- Improvement in peripheral vision, facilitating a better view of your surroundings for better visual threat perception
- Sharper hearing, enabling better auditory threat perception
- Decreased pain perception, allowing you to run, fight, or remain still even if you are wounded
- Sweaty and cold skin, as blood leaves the extremities to focus on major muscle groups involved in running, fighting, and freezing
- Increased heart rate, bringing more oxygen to the major muscle groups involved in responding to threats

It doesn't have to be something as extreme as a bear sighting. We are triggered all the time in our day-to-day lives. To a much smaller extent, our sympathetic nervous system might come on board when:

- Someone taps you on the shoulder when you thought you were alone in a room

- An unsafe driver cuts you off on the freeway

- Your neighbor's large, unleashed dog starts bounding toward you

- You see your child about to have an accident on the playground

- A giant cockroach comes flying at your face

Adults might also experience full-on symptoms of panic when being triggered. This is most likely to happen following a trauma. It might look like a man who was held up at gunpoint at an ATM breaking out into a cold sweat before he even approaches an ATM to deposit a check months later.

I cannot overstate that this stress response is a healthy and adaptive survival instinct that has kept our species going for thousands of years.

So, then, what's the problem?

In people with a trauma history, especially those with active post-traumatic stress symptoms, this protective system can go a bit haywire. Threat can be perceived everywhere, leaving the person feeling constantly on guard or hypervigilant. And for kids, who naturally may have trouble regulating their emotions, things can quickly get out of control. This is an exhausting way to go through life. It means that, in exchange for possibly being more ready to respond to a threat, a child could be less able to pay attention at school or work, engage with friends and family, and be present in day-to-day life.

The key takeaway: Triggers are a normal part of a trauma response and perhaps the most common behavioral change we see in traumatized children. They are automatic, physiological processes that have been present in our biology for centuries, and they help keep us safe. At the same time, triggers can interfere with fundamental aspects of a child's functioning. See Chapter 5 for specific details on how to help your child manage triggers and learn how to calm themselves after experiencing one.

Increased Emotionality and Behavioral Regression

The introduction to this chapter oriented you to the idea that the majority of the behavioral changes you might see in your child after exposure to a potentially traumatic experience are in some way healthy as they aim to protect the self against trauma-related distress. Some of these responses are more effective than others.

The most mature way to go about seeking help from trauma-related distress would be to use words, expressing overwhelming thoughts or feelings and asking directly for what the child needs (for example, "I feel sad on the anniversary of Uncle Ben's car crash. Can we all share our favorite memories of him tonight?"). However, the capacity to do this is elusive even for some of my most self-actualized adult patients, never mind a traumatized child.

The closest some kids can get to this direct verbal expression of feelings and requests for what they need is through displays of increased emotionality. In its mildest form, this can look like increased tearfulness. As it escalates, the emotionality can turn into behavioral regression, such as baby talk or wetting the bed.

Think back to Chapter 3 and what we discussed about attachment. When securely attached babies are feeling distressed, whether it be due to hunger, a dirty diaper, or feelings of being overwhelmed, they will cry out for their primary caregiver and will typically be rewarded by that caregiver's coming to the rescue by soothing them or otherwise addressing their needs.

That tearfulness, whether it comes from an infant or an older child, is essentially sending the same message: I need help. Because so much of the trauma response occurs outside the child's awareness, it's pretty close to impossible to expect children to be able to calmly and confidently use their words to advocate for their needs. They are incredibly distressed, and crying (yes, literally crying) out for help from a trusted caregiver is probably the next healthiest thing they can do if they can't use their words.

If crying doesn't work to garner the support your child needs, there may be an escalation in how the child seeks your support. Perhaps instead of a few tears rolling down a cheek, you'll see a child who cries harder, longer, and sucks his thumb, even though he abandoned that particular self-soothing practice long ago. But just like some mild transient tears, this regression into thumb sucking might just be your son's way of seeking a little extra TLC. Parents might see this and think, "Ugh. He's just using this to get attention. Maybe if I ignore it, it will go away."

Indeed, if you ignore it, it might go away, as parental attention is the number-one driver of child behavior. At the same time, your child's needs will be going unmet. The child who is feeling sad and overwhelmed on the anniversary of his uncle's death will instead be left alone with those feelings, making them feel even more unbearable. With that in mind, it might be more helpful to reframe thoughts like "He's just doing this to get attention—I should ignore this" as "This is how he's telling me he needs a little extra support right now."

While it is normal to be concerned if your happy-go-lucky girl is suddenly crying all the time, or your toddler boy who mastered toilet training is now wetting his pants regularly, please consider these cases of increased emotionality and regression to be a temporary and natural part of the healing process. See Chapter 6 for specific recommendations on how to support your child through these changes.

Minor Misbehavior

Tantrums, whining, back talk, and noncompliance are all examples of what I like to call minor misbehavior. These behaviors are common after a child is exposed to a potentially traumatic event, and

I often emphasize the importance of distinguishing these behaviors from more serious acting out (destruction of property, physical aggression, and the like), which can also occur post–trauma exposure, but will be addressed separately.

Adults often assume that children acting disrespectfully need stricter rules and punishment to help break them of this behavior. While strict rules may indeed shape behavior in a way that is pleasing to caregivers, those rules likely will not meet the need underlying the new behavior. In fact, forcing a traumatized child to change behavior without addressing the core issue can actually make things worse.

A metaphor I often share with parents of traumatized children— that I initially learned in a training for trauma-focused cognitive-behavioral therapy (TF-CBT; see Chapter 11 for more on this approach)—is that coping with trauma is lot like trying to hold an inflated beach ball beneath the water in a pool. After a terrifying experience, it is normal for anyone (child or adult) to want to push down painful thoughts, feelings, and trauma-related memories. But like keeping down a beach ball, it's hard work pushing down these thoughts and feelings—hard work that is essentially impossible to sustain. Like the beach ball, these suppressed thoughts and feelings may come flying out of the water at any time in forceful ways. For kids, this may look like your easygoing boy throwing a tantrum in response to minor annoyances or your sweet-natured girl suddenly talking back to you and ignoring your requests. And like a beach ball, the deeper you try to press those feelings down, the bigger and more sudden the eruption at the end will be.

So, while this minor acting out can be annoying or frustrating, keep in mind that it is likely just a manifestation of your child's defenses failing. Picture the back talk or the tantrum as the moment that everything becomes too much for your child, the moment the beach ball comes flying out of the water. This defiance says less about you or your parenting skills and more about how your child is having a hard time managing overwhelming thoughts and feelings about the trauma. See Chapter 7 for specific recommendations on how you can both support your child through these hard moments and mitigate some of these behaviors.

Withdrawal and Avoidance

If minor misbehaviors are the action of the beach ball flying out of the water, withdrawal is the action of pushing down painful thoughts and feelings that precede this. Of all the behavioral changes that may take place following exposure to a potentially traumatic event, withdrawal is one of the most straightforward. Think about it: If something is causing your daughter intense distress and discomfort, doesn't it make sense that she would want to pull back and avoid it? Like other behavioral changes, withdrawal can be, at least initially, somewhat healthy. A trauma reminder pops up, your child feels horrible and avoids the reminder, and the distress decreases. The child feels better in the short term, but the fear response builds and builds the more the child avoids the reminder—recall the anxiety tiger metaphor from Chapter 2.

While it may be painful to see your child in distress and tempting to let your child withdraw from the things that cause anxiety, this process can exacerbate the trauma symptoms and shrink the child's world. It may seem harmless enough to let it go when your child skips a football game or family dinner. When this becomes a regular practice, however, it can feel impossible to break out of. Even worse, in some children, fear has a tendency to generalize.

Picture Mark, from the beginning of this chapter, who was attacked by a large, aggressive dog while playing in his front yard. At first Mark, who used to love dogs, avoids all large, aggressive dogs of the same breed as the dog that attacked him. Any time he sees a dog like this, he dashes back to the safety of his home. Each time he closes the door behind him, he breathes a sigh of relief. One day a neighbor is walking his medium-sized dog, which is not quite aggressive, but energetic and loud, and has a tendency to playfully jump on the neighborhood kids as a greeting. Mark feels a little uneasy and retreats inside just to be safe. Over time, this pattern of behavior leads to his avoiding all dogs, feeling deeply terrified when one crosses his path. Eventually, he stops playing outside altogether.

Your child is just doing what feels best when he withdraws and avoids, but we know how this can adversely affect the healing process. It can be a complex dance to help support your child in exposing himself to stimuli that remind him of the trauma, while not pushing him too hard. For guidance on this, look to Chapter 8.

Major Misbehavior

As we move up the continuum into more intensive behavioral changes, it becomes increasingly important to seek professional help. While therapy can be helpful in addressing increased emotionality, behavioral regression, withdrawal, and minor acting out, it is not always necessary. For the next set of behavior changes, including major misbehavior and high-risk impulsive behaviors, professional help is strongly advised.

I like to define the line between major acting out and minor misbehavior as the point at which those behaviors begin to jeopardize safety, well-being, and personal property. While both minor and major misbehavior in traumatized children may stem from a need for additional support, major acting out is almost always preceded by intense anger. If your child has displayed multiple incidents of major acting out (say, breaking a sibling's laptop, punching a hole in a wall, kicking the family dog), you probably have a strong reaction of your own to your child's anger! It can be terrifying to see your child act in aggressive, violent, or scary ways. In this situation, many caregivers feel like they need to walk on eggshells around their child, trying their hardest to avoid frustrating them.

Instead of walking on eggshells, it would be more helpful to your child (in the long term) to help them understand where this anger is coming from. As with anything else, there is rarely one explanation, but instead a confluence of factors coming together that result in these volcano-like eruptions. Like the causes of other behavioral changes, issues like sleep impairment, increased irritability, increased negative thoughts and feelings, and struggles to express thoughts and feelings with words all may contribute to a greater prevalence of major acting out. Additionally, a child might act out as an automatic response to feeling triggered.

The current thinking on these symptoms, summarized in 2014 by the Committee on Child Maltreatment Research, Policy, and Practice for the National Research Council, is that untreated childhood trauma may disrupt a child's ability to learn how to successfully regulate emotion, though there are also studies indicating genetic influences may play a role in the development of these symptoms. Additionally, if the child's early trauma exposure included violence and aggression, particularly if this was modeled in the child's home over a long period of time, using violence and aggression to express anger can become normalized. For guidance on how to respond to major acting out, see Chapter 9.

Impulsive Behaviors

In my clinical experience, nothing freaks parents out like a child engaging in risky, impulsive behaviors. I once had a patient who was experiencing severe bullying and had a lot of shame related to the bullying. Her shame was so intense she found it near impossible to tell anyone about her being bullied. She took to impulsively cutting her arms and legs as a way to express that something was wrong without having to put words to her painful experience. One day her parents got a call from the school that a teacher had observed superficial wounds, and they immediately both took off work, picked her up from school, and got the first available appointment with me for a therapy intake. Speaking to me, they were convinced their daughter was mere minutes away from taking her own life. While her parents were right to be alarmed, it was also helpful for them to understand that their daughter's behavior was distinct from suicide and that their daughter could be helped.

Like increased emotionality and behavioral regression, impulsive behaviors including self-injury, drug and alcohol abuse, and high-risk sexual behaviors can sometimes be cries for help, as was the case with the patient described above.

In addition to seeking support, there are a number of other reasons children and adolescents may engage in risky, impulsive behaviors.

One of the healthiest reasons someone might engage in impulsive behaviors is to quiet thoughts about death. Perhaps instead of planning suicide, your teen may intentionally (or unintentionally) open up a hookup app looking for an immediate distraction. Scary? Certainly. Serious? Absolutely. But without a doubt better than the alternative.

Older children and teens might also engage in impulsive behaviors in an attempt to bond with peers who are doing the same. Perhaps all of the girls in your daughter's friend group are carving a symbol into their ankle, and your girl happily does the same to bolster her connection to the group.

Others might do so to help with feeling emotionally numb. Tired of feeling disconnected from their bodies, traumatized kids may race a car or shoplift a trinket in an attempt to feel something.

While there is typically more than one reason someone might engage in impulsive behaviors, research indicates that perhaps the most common function is to help regulate emotional distress. In fact, studies have shown that more than 90 percent of people who engage in nonsuicidal self-injury do so to help ease intense negative thoughts and feelings.

Picture this: Your fourteen-year-old daughter is feeling overwhelmed and distressed after she was asked to testify against a peer who assaulted her. She retreats to her bedroom and feels like she is about to hyperventilate. She is crying and feels helpless to calm herself down. This helpless feeling is the same feeling she experienced during her assault. She goes and grabs the scissors in her desk drawer and makes some shallow cuts on her forearm. Almost immediately, she is able to calm down as she focuses intently on this painful sensation, reclaiming a sense of control in an otherwise spiraling moment.

For information on how to navigate responding to risky, impulsive behaviors, see Chapter 10.

If your child has attempted suicide or admits having thoughts about taking their own life, the child's emotional pain is likely so intense and overwhelming that living feels unbearable. In other instances, a suicide attempt may be the most desperate bid to elicit help from friends or family. In both cases, the important thing to focus on is that this is your child's way of telling you they can't live the way they are anymore.

Something I hear a lot from parents of kids who have attempted suicide in relatively nonlethal ways (like overdosing on three pills of 1 mg of melatonin) is a sense of annoyance that their child is just doing this "to get attention." Here's what I want to say to parents who think this way: Thank goodness your child is communicating to you a need for your attention and support. Regardless of the lethality of your child's attempt, seek therapy and take this attempt seriously. Other than these two recommendations, this book will not cover responding to suicide attempts, as this is something that should always be addressed directly with the child's therapist and/or psychiatrist. Specific resources you can use to help keep your child safe while you connect with professionals can be found on page 211.

The take-home message: Trauma can overwhelm our kids' ability to successfully navigate life. Benign stressors that might have been nothing, or simply a minor annoyance, before trauma exposure can send a child into a seemingly hysterical fit of tears or flying off the handle in a rage. It is important to keep in mind that, regardless of how your child's behaviors have changed, the child is not forever damaged and is not doing this to annoy you. Children who have been exposed to a trauma are coping as best they can, trying to protect themselves from additional trauma or emotional pain, and in each case we as caregivers have a responsibility to respond by providing them with the extra support and attention necessary to help them heal. If you can keep this message in mind, you will be better able to support your child regardless of whatever behavioral changes may pop up, leaving your child feeling more supported and less isolated in grappling with posttraumatic stress.

5

Recognizing
and Responding
to Trauma Triggers

This chapter will walk you through what triggers are, why traumatized kids get triggered, what triggers look like in daily life, and how to respond effectively and best support your children when they experience a trigger. As explained in Chapter 4, trauma triggers are stimuli that pop up and remind our bodies of the scary thing that we have endured. Even if the stressor is long gone, things in your child's everyday environment can bring about sudden physiological changes—faster breathing, sweating, a pounding heart. These changes can reignite many of the trauma symptoms that otherwise might have lessened following a child's original exposure to a potentially traumatic experience, leaving the child feeling panicked and scared.

You may also recall from Chapter 4 that behavioral changes are ways people can protect themselves from trauma-related symptoms. Sometimes these self-protection attempts are relatively healthy coping mechanisms. For example, if a child who was regularly attacked by the same bully felt triggered and ran away each time he sensed this boy's presence, he might be saving himself from another beating. Another student who wasn't as sensitive to his physical proximity to this bully might become the next victim instead.

At the same time, if triggers persist, they can have a negative, limiting impact on your child's life. Think about it: Each day would quickly turn miserable if your body were filled to the limit with stress hormones any time you heard a loud, sudden noise or some otherwise harmless trigger.

This constant triggering likely leads to an increase in other negative thoughts and feelings, and perhaps a tendency to engage in some of the other behavioral changes introduced in Chapter 4 (for example, misbehavior, withdrawal) in order to cope. Helping your child deal with these triggers is an important part of supporting healing and helping the child live a more pleasant life—one that isn't filled with frequent stressors.

Let's take a look at what trauma triggers might actually look like in children and adolescents:

Five-year-old Santi and his mother were in a car accident two months ago. All of the passengers and drivers involved walked away with only minor scrapes and bruises, but Santi has been exhibiting some behavioral changes that worry his mother. He begs her to walk him to school each morning rather than drive. While she typically indulges him in this, one morning, when lightning and thunder fill the sky, she insists on driving him to school. He immediately starts complaining of a headache, and when she moves to gauge his temperature, she finds that his forehead is cool and his brow slick with sweat. He flinches as she fastens him into his car seat and screams when he hears a car honk. His mom yells at him to calm down and tells him to quit being a baby. When they arrive at school, Santi avoids eye contact with his mother. After school, during pickup, Santi's teacher remarks to his mother that he seemed uncharacteristically sullen all morning.

In Santi's case, riding in a car reminded his body of the scary car accident, and hearing a horn honk was an additional trigger. Because

Santi is typically able to avoid exposure to these triggers, his distress is all the more intense on a rainy day when he can't get out of riding in a car. His mother's unthinking response to his being triggered may have brought forth some additional posttraumatic stress symptoms of withdrawal and avoidance, which was then perceived by his teacher as sullenness.

Fourteen-year-old Brittani was at a concert weeks ago where she was accidentally trampled while standing near a mosh pit next to the stage. While her friends were able to help her get up, she was left with a black eye, cracked rib, and painful bruises all over her body. Her injuries healed with proper medical care, and Brittani thought she was fine until she went with her family to her town's fall festival, which was unusually crowded. While waiting in a long line at the cotton candy stand, Brittani started to be overwhelmed by all the people around her. She felt her heart racing as her eyes darted around for a clear path to exit.

For Brittani, the experience of being surrounded by a teeming crowd without an easy escape route reminded her body of her scary experience at the concert.

Twelve-year-old Jacob had a serious bout of food poisoning and had to be hospitalized for twenty-four hours for treatment. During the course of treatment, nursing staff had a hard time starting Jacob's IV line. At first this was because Jacob was dehydrated, making his veins harder to find. As they kept trying to place the IV, he grew frightened and refused to sit still. Ultimately, several staff members had to be called in to restrain him. This terrified Jacob, and one year later his mother has to bribe him with birthday-level gifts to even walk into the doctor's office. Once there, she sees the fear in his eyes. He cannot sit still in the waiting room. He looks as pale as a sheet, and when she grabs his hand to try to comfort him, she finds it ice cold to the touch.

Jacob's scary experience during his hospitalization had stuck with him. His body was trying to warn him and keep him safe from a repeat of the same experience.

How to React Effectively When Your Child Is Triggered

When children experience a trigger, it can be hard to keep in mind that their actions are part of an unconscious, automatic, physiological process and they are not being "too sensitive" or testing your boundaries. There are a number of practices and skills you can utilize to help decrease the frequency and intensity of triggers. Here are some of the basics:

First and Foremost, Remember to Be Empathic and Compassionate

Be Thoughtful

We can all understand why Santi's mother might feel exasperated by her son's trauma response. It's unnerving to hear your child yell from the back seat, perhaps especially so for an adult who was recently in a crash. At the same time, if we thoughtlessly vent this frustration, it could make things worse. In minimizing or dismissing the feelings that come up for a child who feels triggered, a parent could unintentionally shame the child for having a stress response and imply that the child needs to hide his struggles from his parent in the future. Instead of sharing your knee-jerk reaction to your child's trauma response, take a deep breath, slow down, and get thoughtful.

Make the Space

Create room for your children to talk about their feelings (if they want to) and praise them for sharing feelings after the fact. You can make this space by asking questions like "What was that like for you?" or offering statements such as "I noticed you seemed nervous when that dog got a little too close." Brittani's dad might say something to her like "Whew, that line for cotton candy was getting a little tight, huh?"

Be Supportive

After inviting your child to share her feelings, make it clear that you support her. For some children, support might look like a hug; for others, words of encouragement might be best. Experiment with different supportive actions and see which feel the most natural to you and your child. With Jacob, who was triggered by the waiting room of the doctor's office, his mom might offer support by saying things like "I'm right here with you" and "I won't leave your side."

Normalize Feeling Scared

Don't feel like you need to act stoic all the time. If certain things scare you, it's okay to share that with your child in a developmentally appropriate way. If you're nervous about an upcoming presentation at work, say so. Santi's mom might share with him that she felt a little nervous getting behind the wheel again for the first time after their accident.

When the Basics Aren't Cutting It

If you've mastered these basics, and your child is still having frequent, intense trauma triggers, therapeutic support is indicated. In between therapy sessions, consider the following tips to help your child maximize the therapy experience and feel supported at home.

Develop a Routine

Sticking to a schedule is one way you can help decrease stress and increase comfort for your traumatized child. Triggers are often things that pop up unexpectedly, and having a structured day will cut down on the likelihood of this sort of experience. Additionally, children who know what to expect from their day will feel more in control and better able to make plans.

Play Detective

Your child may not make the connection between a past traumatic event and current distress, but that doesn't mean you can't make sense of it. If you notice your child is triggered, make a note of it. If it is something that happens frequently, keep a log.

I once worked with a parent who made an offhand comment about how her daughter's typically affable attitude would inexplicably shift to doom and gloom whenever she took a moment's glance at her phone on Tuesday evenings. In therapy, we tried to explore what was different about Tuesdays compared to other nights of the week. When we broke down her week, the girl shared that Tuesday nights were school football games, which she used to enjoy attending before being sexually assaulted by one of the players. She shared that after the assault, she did not feel comfortable going to the games anymore. Not only was she resentful of missing out on a fun social outing, but she also felt betrayed by her friends who still went to enjoy the games. She would inevitably become triggered later that night when her social media feed was inundated with pictures of her friends and the players, including the boy who assaulted her, having fun. While this triggering was outside of the girl's awareness, if you as her parent can observe these patterns, you can plan extra support for these times in advance and provide helpful information to your child's therapist.

Develop a Secret Code

I once had a patient who was physically assaulted by a neighbor. She was left with broken bones, and the police conducted a lengthy investigation, but the case was closed with no repercussions for the alleged perpetrator. My patient would frequently see her attacker at the neighborhood drugstore or market and experienced panic attacks when this happened. When her mother first observed these panic attacks, she could not understand what was happening. The mother's attempts at calming her down inadvertently drew more attention to the daughter, who would have rather had her panic attack crouched in the corner behind the canned goods display than have her mother dragging her to the front exit of the store. In therapy, we devised a secret code word the girl could use if she ever saw this boy in public again. Your code word could be something simple, like *tomato*. Just pick a word or signal your child can use to get your attention. Then the two of you can devise a plan to get somewhere your child feels safer. If you are somewhere that feels safe and your child is still triggered by something (say, loud fireworks going off in the neighborhood), it will still be helpful for your child to only have to utter one word rather than explain the nuanced, uncomfortable process going on in her body.

Biohacking

For decades, therapists have relied on strategies that help people better regulate their emotions in times of stress. These well-established practices are known as *relaxation training skills* in the therapy world, but it is also fun to think about them as *biohacking*. This loaded term has been steadily gaining popularity over the past few years, but at its core it refers to manipulating the brain or body to your own benefit. There are some simple yet surprisingly effective grounding and relaxation techniques you can teach your children to help them "biohack" and activate their parasympathetic (or cooldown) response when they are in the midst of a trigger.

Some important caveats: First, keep in mind that not every technique will resonate with every kid. You should aim to find one to two techniques that your child enjoys and can easily utilize when needed. Second, no one is good at learning a new skill while being triggered. The following skills are meant to be learned when a child is feeling safe and calm, and practiced regularly, so that when these tools are needed in a crisis your child will have a set of go-to, tried-and-true methods. On this note, it might be more helpful to your child to go to a safe location before employing the skills. For example, with my patient who saw her alleged perpetrator in a grocery store, it would be more helpful to get into her mom's car or back to the family home and then use these skills to help self-regulate.

Finally, the effectiveness of these skills is not just about technique. It's about building a connection between parent and child. These strategies have been proven to be helpful even when used alone, but the benefits increase significantly when practiced together with someone a child is securely attached to. With that in mind, here are some of the most accessible grounding and relaxation strategies:

- **5-4-3-2-1**: This skill helps children engage with their senses, which can help bring them to the present moment. When we are in the present moment, we are not ruminating about the past or worrying about the future, which is often a big source of distress for children and adults alike. This skill works for children, adolescents, and adults. Use the instructions below to guide your practice of this activity:

  1. First, instruct your child to look around and identify five things they can **see**. The first time you introduce this skill, it could be helpful to model this (for example, "I see your green shoes, the glass picture frame, my old teacup, the cactus plant, and our fuzzy rug").

  2. Next, four things the child can **feel** ("I feel my soft T-shirt, my damp hair on my shoulders, the glasses resting on the bridge of my nose, and this mosquito bite on my knee").

  3. Then three things the child can **hear** ("I hear the sound of my voice, a car honking outside, and the hum of the air conditioner").

  4. Two things the child can **smell** ("I am lifting up and smelling this candle, and I can also smell my perfume").

  5. Finally, one thing the child can **taste** ("I can taste the toothpaste I used this morning").

These five steps are easy to remember, and you can prompt your child to go through them almost anywhere at any time when the child is triggered: in the car, at home, outdoors, in a restaurant or store, at a relative's or friend's home. Once your child can recall the steps without your assistance, this is also a great skill he could use on his own. I have many young patients who silently practice 5-4-3-2-1 at their desks after a classroom trigger or when out with friends if they feel panicked during a social outing.

 • **Body scans:** Like 5-4-3-2-1, body scans can help us connect to the present moment, where feelings of intense distress are likely to be lessened. This is another skill that can be used with all ages. Adolescents may not be as interested in having you read a script to them while they lie down (see more on teens in the box below), but they can easily stream a body scan script from the Internet and do this by themselves. A sample script for a body scan that you can read out loud

---

What If You Get Pushback from Your Teenager?

Practicing relaxation training skills with a triggered child packs a one-two punch: your proximity and presence can bring a sense of connection and groundedness to their inner chaos, *and* the skills can help activate the body's natural relaxation response. At the same time, teens are less likely than younger children to want to engage with parents in this way, even when they are feeling triggered. As explained in Chapter 10, this is a part of the natural growing-up process where children seek more independence. Here's my advice to the parent of a teen who rebuffs a parent's attempt at practicing one of these skills together: Don't force it. If your child is open to listening to a body scan or progressive muscle relaxation script alone, take this as a win. The more you try to force something on teenagers, the more they may push back. This pushback could look like an explicit rejection or, in a more compliant teen, inner resentment of you and what you're trying to teach.

so your child can follow is on the facing page. If you find that the body scan is helpful to your child, consider recording yourself reading the script so that it can be used even if you are not immediately available. Bedtime is an ideal time for practicing body scans, so that your child can easily lie down and get comfortable and won't be exposed to many distractions.

• **Diaphragmatic breathing**: Diaphragmatic breathing is one of my favorite go-tos as a therapist. When children are triggered, their breathing speeds up. Instead of deep, relaxing breaths, they are likely to start breathing rapid, shallow breaths into their chest, which serves to further activate the sympathetic nervous system/fight–flight–freeze response. Instead of helping them calm down, this quickened breathing actually makes them more anxious. There are two simple rules for effective diaphragmatic breathing:

1. First, it's essential for your child to breathe in through the nose and out through the mouth. This is important because when we are anxious we often take in more oxygen than we expel. Have you ever seen someone hyperventilate when nervous? That's exactly what's happening and why in old movies you might see a nervous child breathing into a paper bag (to cut down on oxygen intake). But if we breathe in through the nose and out through the mouth, we are reversing that, putting out just a little more oxygen than we are taking in.

2. Second, your child should breathe into the diaphragm— located above the belly button, below the chest—rather than the chest. You can walk the child through this by resting an object (a stuffed animal or tissue box will work just fine) on the child's diaphragm. You want to see the object rise with each inhalation and fall with each exhalation.

It could be especially helpful to model this before your child attempts it. Try to really exaggerate the object rising and falling so your kid gets the picture. This is another skill that's great for all ages. It's

BODY SCAN SCRIPT

"Start by sitting in a chair or lying on a couch or bed. Leave your hands at your sides or in your lap and close your eyes. Take a deep breath in through your nose . . . and out through your mouth. Bring your attention to your hands. Notice how your hands feel. Imagine taking a deep breath in through your nose and sending that breath all the way to the tips of your fingers. Exhale slowly through your mouth.

"Move your attention up to your arms. Notice any feelings or sensations you have in your arms. Again, take a deep breath in through your nose and visualize sending that breath into your arms. Then give a nice long exhale through your mouth.

"Next, check in with your head, neck, and shoulders. What feelings do you have in your head, neck, and shoulders? Envision taking a deep breath in through your nose and filling up your entire head, face, down to your neck and then your shoulders. Exhale through your mouth.

"Move your attention to your core. What feelings do you notice in your chest, your diaphragm, your stomach? Take a deep breath in through your nose and picture sending your breath to your core. Exhale through your mouth, nice and slow.

"Now let's check in with our legs and knees. What sensations do you notice in your thighs, knees, and lower legs? Take a deep breath in through your nose and visualize sending your breath down to the bottom of your legs. Exhale through your mouth.

"Finally, check in with your feet and toes. Connect with any sensations in your feet and toes. Take a big breath in through your nose and envision sending it down your legs to your feet and the tips of your toes. Exhale a nice slow breath through your mouth."

typically the first one I teach to patients because it resonates with most people—I've even had adult patients tell me it was effective in helping them birth a child! If you are teaching your child diaphragmatic breathing, you might make this a nightly practice to help your child wind down before bed. When first practicing this new skill, try to start with one minute. As your child gets more comfortable with this method of breathing, you can increase the time to two or three minutes.

Adolescents may appreciate the guidance for diaphragmatic breathing on various smartphone apps aimed at meditation or relaxation. The Apple iWatch even has a built-in breathing app that can help guide your child through the practice. For a list of relaxation training resources, flip to page 209.

• **Mindful walking**: In our day-to-day lives, walking is something we treat as the means to an end: transportation. But if we incorporate mindfulness into our walking practice, it can become a wonderful coping skill. As with the other relaxation training skills covered here, it is ideal to get your child familiar with these practices before they need them amid a trigger. You might do mindful walking twice a week with your child when he gets home from school. Children of all ages can enjoy mindful walking with parents, siblings, and friends. Older children may also appreciate this practice in solitude. Here are some tips to start mindful walking:

- Ask your child how their body feels. Heavy and sluggish or light and energetic? Feeling any sunshine or raindrops? A cool breeze?

- Think together about how the act of taking steps feels.

- What can your child see? Maybe a house with a unique door? Inspiring trees? Interesting road signs?

- What does your child hear? Rustling leaves? Honking horns?

- Any smells?

- **Progressive muscle relaxation**: One part of our bodies' natural stress response is for our muscles to tense up. Progressive muscle relaxation involves tensing and relaxing different muscle groups to lead to a deeper state of muscle relaxation. It could be helpful to follow a script like the one on page 94 with imagery for children ages three through eight. Older children might prefer to use an app or stream a video that walks them through it.

Like 5-4-3-2-1, it would be easy for a child familiar with progressive muscle relaxation to use this skill when triggered away from a supportive caregiver. Just picture a panicked student tightening his abs while seated after being triggered during a lecture or a jittery girl pushing her toes down to the bottom of her sleeping bag when triggered while away at a sleepover.

Progressive muscle relaxation is easy to practice at home—when decompressing after school, taking a break from homework, or at bedtime—and because the sequence can be completed in as little as five minutes children may be able to do it unobtrusively in a variety of settings, like while riding in a carpool, shuffling in the hallway between classes, or at the cafeteria lunch table.

For adolescents who might not be as receptive to this type of script, progressive muscle relaxation can still be completed by going through the major muscle groups of the body, tensing them for several seconds, and releasing them.

- **Visualization:** Visualization combines some of the best parts of grounding techniques and relaxation exercises. You can help guide your child to a peaceful, calming place. When your child is imagining this place, inquire about the child's senses. Your older child or teen may be less receptive to being questioned about how they visualize their senses but could be prompted to touch base with what they smell, hear, feel, see, and taste via a script or recording.

Therapists often rely on completed scripts to help guide a child patient. One that I have used is on page 95.

PROGRESSIVE MUSCLE RELAXATION SCRIPT

"Imagine it's nighttime and you're about to brush your teeth with your favorite toothpaste. The tube has been running low for a few nights, and you know you're going to need to squeeze really hard to get the last bit out to brush your teeth tonight. Take your left hand and squeeze it! Squeeze it as hard as you can. You see a tiny little bit coming up out of the top; squeeze even harder. There it goes—that's a good amount; you can relax. [repeat with right hand]

"Now let's pretend we are playing charades, and you just picked the word *sour*. How can we show everyone what sour looks like? Let's scrunch up our faces as tight as we can, like when we suck on a sour candy. Ooh, scrunch your face up tight, it looks like someone might be about to guess it! Scrunch it tight, tight, tight! And you did it, you really showed everyone what sour looks like.

"Now imagine you're lying down in the grass on a sunny day. All of a sudden, you hear barking, and [family dog's name] comes bounding out the back door, rushing over to you excitedly. You don't have time to get up or move out of the way, and he's about to land right on your stomach. Tighten up your stomach muscles as hard as you can so he doesn't smush you! Oh, here he comes. Front paws on you, pounce. Keep it tight. Now back paws on you. Stay tight; you're doing great! And . . . he's off; you can relax.

"Now you're standing on a warm, sandy beach. Try to bury your feet in the sand without using your hands or any tools. That's right, tighten up your legs and push those toes deep into the wet sand. Feel your toes sink down and keep pushing. There they—oh—your toes are practically covered! Push some more. You're doing great. And . . . you can step out and relax."

VISUALIZATION SCRIPT FOR A YOUNG CHILD

"Let's get started by finding a safe place to lie down and take a deep breath in through the nose and out through the mouth . . . Let's imagine a beach with warm white sands. As you look out to the water, you see large turquoise waves, so clear they look like glass . . . There's not a soul in sight . . . As you look up to the sky, there are no clouds out today; all you see is a magnificent blue . . . You feel the warm, soft sand underneath your toes . . . There's a slight breeze, which lightly blows your hair back . . . You breathe in through your nose and smell the salty ocean air . . . You watch as the waves crash, again and again, and rise up on the shore, stopping just before your feet."

Adolescents might be more receptive to listening to a sample script on their own. The Resources at the back of the book include apps your teen can use (including Calm and Wellemental) with you or alone for a more structured way to practice these skills.

Using New Skills to Respond to Triggers in Daily Life

These skills may sound great in theory, but there are a few practical considerations to reflect on before implementing them in everyday life. Santi's mom might introduce 5-4-3-2-1 when they get home from school. Remember, these skills should not be taught in the midst of a trigger. Santi wouldn't be capable of participating or learning something new in the heat of the moment, and neither would your child. When a child is triggered, their thinking brain goes offline. But after school, when Santi is calm if a bit sullen, could be a wonderful opportunity to connect, validate his feelings, and teach a new skill.

Here's what it might look like:

MOM: I love our special walks to school, and it's too bad it was too rainy for us to walk today.

SANTI: I don't like the car. I only like to walk with you to school.

MOM: I hear you—you and I would both rather walk to school. It looked like you were feeling pretty scared this morning in the car?

SANTI: Yeah, I just don't like it. We could get into an accident.

MOM: I hear you, sweetie. It feels scary to you. It's normal to worry about accidents after what happened with our silver car. When I'm feeling scared, I do something called 5-4-3-2-1 to help my body relax. First I try, really fast, to think of five things I see. Right now, I see my white cup, your light-up shoes, my big purse, the green grass through the window, and our round breakfast table. What are five things you see right now?

SANTI: I see my backpack, your blue glasses, the floor, my hands, and that plate.

MOM: Nice work naming things you see! Then I pay attention to my body to find four things I can feel. Right now I feel the soft cotton on my dress, my bracelet moving around my wrist, my braces rubbing against my lips, and my snuggly socks on my feet. What are four things you can feel?"

SANTI: I feel my ant bites, they're itchy . . . and my shorts, my shirt, and my new shoes.

MOM: Great examples of things you can feel! Next, I listen quietly for three things I can hear. Right now I hear the hum of the air conditioner, I hear our neighbor mowing his lawn, and I hear some crickets outside chirping. What are three things you can hear?

SANTI: I hear the lawnmower too. And the garbage truck and the air conditioner too.

MOM: After that I sniff around for two things I can smell. Right now I can smell the flowers we have on our table and the scent of your shampoo. What about you?

SANTI: I can't smell my shampoo. I smell your shampoo and the flowers too.

MOM: We smelled similar things. Last up I swish my tongue around my mouth and see if I can taste one thing. Right now I can taste some gum I was chewing on the way to pick you up. What about you?

SANTI: I don't taste anything.

MOM: Yeah, that one can be hard. Do you want to taste a mint? You did a great job with 5-4-3-2-1, and we can use it anytime we are feeling nervous, worried, or scared to help our bodies feel calmer.

Eight days later, another rainy day hits and Santi must ride to school. As his mom is pulling out of their driveway, she sneaks a glance at him in her rearview mirror. Santi is chewing on his lip and getting twitchy. She senses he is one sudden brake or car honk away from a full-blown freakout.

MOM: Santi, you look nervous.

SANTI: (*No response.*)

MOM: I get that riding in a car can feel scary after our accident. How about we try 5-4-3-2-1. I'll go first, I see . . . What about you?

Jacob's mom might try to brainstorm something fun for the two of them to do together after the doctor's appointment. Perhaps Jacob is a big ice cream fan, and Mom agrees that the two of them can hit up his favorite spot afterwards. When she notices Jacob getting antsy in the waiting room, she might come up with her own visualization, based on the ice cream shop. Here's what that might sound like:

"Okay, let's close our eyes and picture ourselves at the Creamery . . . You can see the long white counter with buckets and buckets of ice cream . . . Hazelnut, Birthday Cake, Jamocha Almond Fudge . . . they all look so wet and creamy . . . And then all the toppings! Oh, they look great tonight. There's the bright rainbow sprinkles, and the gooey gummy bears, oh, and your favorite—the chocolate chips . . . They look extra crunchy tonight . . . At the end of the counter you see the freezer . . . Frost icing over the freezer window, and you know the delicious ice cream cakes are sitting safe inside . . . Take a deep breath in through your nose and smell those yummy waffle cones . . . ahhhh. You can hear the sounds of kids laughing. Everyone's feeling so happy to be there."

With an older child like Brittani, her father might anticipate that going to any future crowded event might be a little anxiety provoking for her. To prepare her, he might say something like "Who knows how crowded this family reunion will be? If you feel yourself starting to get nervous, you can give me a nod. We could go off by the restrooms and do some watch breathing together or grab a snack outside." Brittani may not respond to this, but rest assured that even if she doesn't acknowledge her father's outreach attempt, she heard it. If he later notices her panicked and scanning for an exit, all he might need to do is make eye contact with her, motion to his watch, and shrug his shoulders inquisitively, suggesting to her he's on standby if she needs some support in calming herself down. This subtle and casual approach is more likely to be well received by teens than the structured, hand-holding approach offered by Santi's mom.

The greater the distress of your child, the harder it will be to implement any of these skills. That's why it's ideal for Santi's mom to implement this skill when he is mildly or moderately triggered by riding in the car, instead of waiting for a full-blown meltdown after a blaring honk. But what about when you encounter your child in such intense distress that they can't focus with you on one of these grounding activities? Think, for example if Santi's mom were to get rear-ended on the way to school. In these cases, recognize that the best thing you can do to help your child is to offer your close physical proximity and full attention (as long as this is safe). Stay with them until they calm down. Don't worry about trying to implement a skill in these moments—your calming presence is more powerful than any relaxation skill.

The take-home message: The human body is a fascinating structure. As a psychologist, I'm always surprised to see the ways our mind works unconsciously to help protect us. When people are triggered, that is their mind and body working in tandem to help keep them safe, but like a well-meaning, overengaged parent, it can overwhelm and undermine even the most well-adjusted survivor of trauma. Use the skills in this chapter to confidently guide your child through triggers, acknowledging they are a natural, normal response *and* there are things the two of you can do together to help the child feel better.

PART III

Responding to Behavioral Changes

6

What to Do When Your Child Becomes More Emotional and Less Mature

In my clinical practice I've had the privilege of working with patients who put their lives on the line as an everyday part of their jobs—SWAT officers, hostage negotiators, Coast Guard rescue swimmers. Over their careers they've built the physical skills and mental fortitude to face down gunmen and run headfirst into a hurricane. By any objective measure, they are some of the toughest people I have ever met. But the insidious nature of posttraumatic stress, whether or not it is related to their job, presents them with a challenge they're unprepared to handle.

Surviving and overcoming trauma can be hard and messy, even for adults with careers straight out of G.I. Joe. So imagine how difficult it can be for someone who is still playing with action figures. Growing kids already have enough trouble controlling their emotions, and the addition of a traumatic event—whether a car crash, physical abuse, or contracting a deadly illness—only makes things worse.

Time and again, I've seen parents respond with alarm when their easygoing, well-adjusted child occasionally starts breaking down following a trauma. This is not surprising. You know your child has had a distressing experience and is still going through it. But that doesn't mean you know how to respond when a typically mundane drive to school suddenly becomes filled with tears or your quick-to-laugh child is now easily angered. It can be difficult to see your formerly robust child start to act "needy" or lacking in resilience. How will your child get along in the world without the strength and equanimity he used to have?

As with other aspects of the response to being traumatized that we've discussed, this emotionality is a normal part of the healing process. It can even be a healthy, adaptive approach to dealing with distress. If your child is acting "needy," it is only because they *need* more support.

A child who has been through a traumatizing experience is crying out—often literally—for connection. Remember, if your child comes to you when upset and cries to you, that says something wonderful about your attachment relationship. It says that you are your child's safe place, where your child can go in times of distress to get the soothing the child needs to heal.

Seeing your child seemingly out of control may make you feel uncomfortable, but emotion expressed outward is far better than what happens when kids bury their distress. Kids who can't cry for help might learn instead to withdraw and avoid their feelings, in the worst cases turning to drugs or alcohol to numb the emotions or even to suicidal behavior.

To revisit the beach ball metaphor from Chapter 4, the kids who exhibit increased emotionality as part of their trauma are those who allow their beach balls to bob on the surface, clear as day for you to see. Those children who feel like they can't express their emotional pain are pushing their beach ball under the water, suffering in silence, until their distress inevitably pops up in one of many different, less adaptive ways.

Some therapists may refer to a display of increased emotionality as "regression." Classically, *regression* refers to a return to earlier stages of development. It's a common defense mechanism that people of all ages use when under intense stress. In children, it can show up as crying and fussing, thumb sucking, bedwetting, and fear of separation from parents, despite these children having long matured past those developmental stages. You have probably seen your child display regression at other times too. Perhaps with the addition of a younger sibling to the family or when starting school for the first time, your little one acted in ways that were typical of someone considerably younger. All of these regressions can be part of normal, natural healing.

Despite this, many parents are unnerved by developmental regressions. Understandably so. Behavioral and developmental milestones are often hard won. How many pairs of ruined pants and stained carpets paved the path to a potty-trained child? It can feel devastating to see that progress suddenly undone. You might even worry that regression will put your kids off track for the rest of their lives, derailing their growth and setting them behind their peers for the rest of their lives.

Let me assure you this is absolutely not the case.

I once treated a seven-year-old girl—with five years of successful toilet usage under her belt—who defecated in her pants a handful of times after an adverse event. She was the only child of two parents who were beside themselves when this happened after she had experienced horrific sexual abuse by her piano teacher. Before they came to see me, they were tempted to pull her from her school and enroll her in a special needs program for children with cognitive struggles. I convinced them to table this idea while we started regular individual therapy for the girl, as well as extra support and coaching for her parents in how to respond to her regression. After a few months of treatment, she was not only using the toilet properly again but was excelling in school and provided damning testimony against her alleged abuser in court.

It may be helpful to think of regression as a signal that your child is struggling to manage his emotional experience and needs more support. Regression is a nonverbal, maybe even unconscious, communication.

Keep in mind too that kids are generally pretty motivated to move forward—rather than backward—in their development. Think back to when your son first learned to tie his shoelaces. After he mastered the skill, did he still want you to tie his shoes? More likely, he was tying not only his own shoes but his little brother or sister's as well, eager to show off his new bow-tying prowess. All this is to say that you should not worry if your little one is taking a few steps back—this is in all likelihood just a sign, again, that the child needs more support.

A caveat: While I can't emphasize enough that regression signals a need for more support and that in response you should provide that additional support, I do not mean that there are no limits to the amount and type of support you should give. Sometimes behavioral regression endures, despite the support you're providing. The most common example I see of this is children who insist on sleeping in their parents' bed after a scary experience. This can be tricky to navigate. On the one hand, we want to give our children that extra support and comfort. At the same time, boundaries around sleep are important, and we don't want to inadvertently send the message that the child's bedroom is somehow unsafe. Generally speaking, room sharing is typically okay for a *brief* period (that is, for a couple of weeks immediately following an adverse event). But parents need to be clear that they are room sharing to give their child extra love, not because the child's room is somehow unsafe or something might happen to the child in the night if their parents aren't there to provide protection. If your child has been sleeping in your bed for a while, see page 139 for a brief plan to gently and gradually decreasing bed sharing or room sharing until your child is again sleeping through the night in her own room without parental assistance.

Whether your child is simply more tearful or trying to sleep in your bed every night, there are several psychological principles that can help guide the most supportive, helpful way you can respond to your vulnerable child.

Talk about It

When I meet with parents dealing with a child overwhelmed by emotion, I often find myself offering up one of my favorite *Star Trek* quotes.

No, it isn't "Beam me up, Scotty" or "Make it so." The quote is "How do you feel?"

The line comes from a scene in which the brilliant Spock tests his mind by subjecting himself to the most difficult questions his computer can summon. He answers all of the trivia questions about science, technology, and philosophy perfectly, demonstrating the brilliance of his logical Vulcan brain. But Spock is also half human, so the computer asks him how he feels. After all, there is little else that shows the strength and health of a human mind like the ability to answer the question "How do you feel?"

We've acknowledged it's very hard for kids—especially traumatized ones—to put words to their painful experience. However, children who can cry to express feelings are closer to using their words than kids who have no idea what they're feeling. When feelings are close to the surface, it means children are in touch with them. All we need to do is help provide the language for children to express their inner experience.

The ultimate goal is for your child to be able to answer the same question the computer posed to Spock and simply respond, "I'm feeling really overwhelmed/sad/lonely/scared."

You might have learned growing up that the magic word is *please.* But when you're trying to help your kid open her emotional door, the magic words are "How are you feeling?" This simple phrase can be a literal open sesame for a child to turn her emotions into words.

But beware: Repeating the same question over and over again might feel grating to you and your child.

Make Talking about Feelings Routine

To get around the risk of annoying, invasive questions, one thing I recommend to all families is making a daily ritual out of talking about feelings. This typically fits into a family's routine around dinnertime. In families with young children, parents could go around the dinner table with everyone taking a turn sharing something that made them feel "warm and fuzzy" and something that made them feel "cold and prickly" that day. Parents share their experience too. For an adult, a "warm, fuzzy" feeling might be expressed as something like "I felt proud when my boss gave me a compliment after my big presentation today," and an example of a "cold, prickly" feeling might be "I felt annoyed and disgusted when I accidentally stepped in Fluffy's poop on our porch." If your child is not receptive to this around dinnertime, try incorporating it as part of the bedtime routine. Most little ones will do anything to earn extra parental engagement when they are winding down for the night.

Modeling these verbal expressions of emotions normalizes talking about thoughts and feelings and gives your child a nice template for doing it.

With older children, "warm, fuzzy" and "cold, prickly" may sound a little babyish, so change up the language. You might each share your rose (something that made you feel good), thorn (something that didn't feel good), and your bud (something you're feeling excited about or looking forward to). With teens, you might just call this "highs and lows" or have a less structured way of talking about your days.

Watch for Opportunities to Put Emotions into Words

You don't have to wait for dinnertime to facilitate talking about thoughts and feelings with your child. Any time you notice a strong emotion pop up in your child (for example, your five-year-old daughter accidentally knocks over her stack of dominoes she'd been working on for the better part of an hour and looks furious), attend to it. Saying something like "Oh no! Your dominoes fell before you were ready— that would make me feel so frustrated! Grr!" may feel supportive (and validating; see the following section) to her and open up the space for her to share those feelings of frustration with you. With very young children, this practice also helps them begin to develop their vocabulary for putting words to their experience.

The goal here is not necessarily to get kids talking about their thoughts and feelings related to the trauma. Discussing feelings like terror, sadness, and all the overwhelming sensations that come from trauma can be too much for dinner conversation and may be better suited for therapy or at least more private conversations. Also, try not to assume your child has overwhelming feelings of fear that need to be processed. As you may recall from Chapter 2, most children who are exposed to a potentially traumatic event do not go on to develop debilitating trauma symptoms.

Rather, the goal is to nurture and grow your child's comfort with using words to express their inner experience. Instead of hoping for insight into your child's trauma, you should be satisfied to hear how, for example, your daughter felt angry when a classmate stole her pencil at school. Your child has to crawl before being able to walk.

The great part of this process is that not only does it clue you in to your child's world, but it also invites your child to be reflective about his own feelings and gives him everyday experience in talking about his inner thoughts.

These conversations also give you a great opportunity to practice the next skill: validation.

Validation

Fifteen-year-old Tom had been looking forward to his family's annual summer vacation at the state park for months. He had been talking all spring about how excited he was that this would be the first year he'd be allowed to drive an ATV on his own. A few weeks before the family was set to leave on their trip, Tom's friend Terrance was in a horrible jet ski accident and ended up paralyzed. Tom was really shaken up by this and mentioned to his parents he did not want anyone in their family to ride ATVs on the upcoming trip. His father, in an attempt to comfort and reassure Tom, replied, "Don't worry, kiddo.

Everything's going to be fine, and you're going to have a blast driving through the park's course!" Tom clenched his jaw and stormed off, without responding to his father.

What went wrong?

In Tom's mind, his concerns about his family's well-being had been dismissed. Rather than attempt to earnestly engage with his father and give him feedback about how that felt, a teenage boy is much more likely to deflect with avoidance and suppression (like Tom has), sarcasm, or even aggression.

So often, well-meaning, competent parents will try to comfort their teary child with a "Don't cry, sweetheart," "Don't worry," or "Everything is fine," whether their child has just skinned a knee or is more sensitive to a trauma trigger after exposure to a potentially traumatic event. These parents' hearts are in the right places—they just want to comfort their child—but they may be inadvertently making it harder for their child to connect with them.

But what's so bad about offering up one of these easy comforts?

It can be a form of minimization, a psychological term for denying or downplaying the significance of a feeling or an event. While you're trying to provide comfort, your child might be getting the message that the potentially traumatic event was actually no big deal and there is something wrong with him for feeling so intensely about it. Over the course of his life, he may internalize your message that "everything is all right" when in fact it is not.

So how best to respond to an increasingly emotional child? My first go-to is validation.

Validation is another tool that started in the therapy office but can also be applied as a parenting practice. In the context of therapy, it refers to the recognition that a patient's thoughts and feelings are legitimate and make sense. So too in the parenting realm: Your child's thoughts and feelings are valid.

The practice is utilized in all types of therapy, but perhaps most notably in dialectical behavior therapy (DBT), a treatment that emphasizes skill acquisition in mindfulness, tolerating distress, interpersonal effectiveness, and regulating emotions—realms where traumatized children and adolescents sometimes struggle.

The idea behind validation is that when children are struggling with uncomfortable thoughts or feelings, especially if they are sensitive or already vulnerable, they can easily become overwhelmed. But if someone—a therapist or a parent—can intervene and communicate that what they are thinking or feeling is okay, it can feel less overwhelming. This helps children feel less alone, better able to tolerate distressing thoughts and feelings, and more capable of regulating their emotions in the long term.

If you take away one lesson from this book, it should be that life is tough enough for kids—and things only grow more complicated after they experience something terrifying. Your task as a parent is to connect with your child so that the child doesn't feel alone in the scary emotional chaos that inevitably follows a trauma.

So how do you validate your child?

Marsha Linehan, the creator of DBT, identified six levels of validation that can be applied to validating your traumatized child. Consider how you might use the spirit of these six levels in validating your child:

- **Pay attention:** When your child is expressing an intense emotion, put your phone down. Stop making a mental grocery list. Give the child your undivided attention. Often parents are uncomfortable with expressions of intense emotion—something that probably stems from their own childhood and how their parents responded to their intense distress. If this trepidation toward emotion feels familiar to you, remind yourself that intense feelings aren't a bad thing. They are just children's way of letting you know they need more support.

- **Provide accurate reflections:** You may recall active listening (also known as reflections) from Chapter 3. This is also an important part of validation. In review, try to put words to what your child is expressing. Don't mimic the child; just rephrase what the child is saying or expressing in your own words.

- **Guess at what hasn't been said aloud:** Your child may not be sure what she's feeling, and by taking a guess you're showing her you are trying to understand her. You might also be helping her make sense of what thoughts or feelings are underlying her behavior.

- **Understand your child's behavior in terms of the child's trauma history:** Show that you see the connection between the child's trauma responses and their underlying trauma experience.

- **Normalize emotional reactions:** Strong, intense emotions can feel isolating. It helps to know that anyone in a similar situation could feel that way.

- **Exhibit radical genuineness:** Really try to relate to and understand your child's strong emotions. Perhaps think back to a time you felt intensely about something.

Depending on how Tom, whose friend was paralyzed in an accident, responds to validation, one simple validating "I hear you—it feels scary to you" might be enough. Other times, using each of these levels of reflection can evolve naturally and feel appropriate. Consider this sample exchange between Tom and his father:

TOM: I don't want anyone riding ATVs.

DAD: [Offering a reflection] You want us to skip over the ATV rides this year. (*pauses for response*)

TOM: That's what I said.

DAD: [Taking a guess at what Tom hasn't said aloud] Feels a little scary?

TOM: Yeah.

DAD: [Trying to understand fear in context of Tom's history] I guess that makes sense, huh, with what you saw happen to Terrance.

TOM: Yeah. And that could happen to any of us. Just get paralyzed or even die. It's just not worth it.

DAD: [Trying to normalize his feelings] I totally get that. You know, I bet anyone who saw an accident like that would want to try to keep his family away from jet skis and ATVs.

TOM: Yeah, I just want everyone to be safe and have a good time.

DAD: [Exhibiting radical genuineness] I hear that . . . actually, before you were born, I got into a horrible accident in my old truck and didn't want to get back behind the wheel for weeks. Those kinds of things can really shake a person up.

TOM: For real.

DAD: Well, I hear you and I get it. You don't have to ride an ATV if you don't want to. We can talk to the rest of the family about what makes sense for them, but I think you're right that we should at least look into some safety precautions so that everyone can feel good about keeping themselves safe.

A conversation like this will help Tom feel heard and respected, improving his relationship with his father. Also, instead of avoiding his feelings (pushing down his beach ball), he'll be sharing them with a validating attachment figure, meaning his fear response should subside, at least a bit.

But what if you can't understand why your child is feeling the need for support? Say Tom's friend never had a life-threatening accident, and Tom was simply fearful of getting back on his ATV after what appeared to them to be a small fender bender. Tom's parents don't think an accident that minor warrants his strong anti-ATV stance. My advice if you find yourself in this situation: Remind yourself that any feeling is okay. Your understanding of your child's inner experience is not a litmus test of validity. In validating these feelings, Tom's parents ensure that he is not alone with them and he will have support. Without this, his feelings may swell in intensity and his discomfort may grow. His parents and the rest of his family can still ride their ATVs, but if they go about it in a way that acknowledges Tom's fears rather than dismissing them, he will be better able to tolerate his distress.

Physical Touch

In addition to using your words to comfort your child, you can use your physical presence. A simple hug, pat on the back, or shoulder rub can go a long way. It starts early. Several studies have found that preterm newborn babies who received massage *for just five to ten days* gained up to 48 percent more weight than premature infants who received the standard protocol of care in the hospital.

In fact, the absence of physical touch can be traumatizing. Recall what we discussed in Chapter 2 about reactive attachment disorder. Sometimes children raised in orphanages or overly crowded foster homes do not receive emotional support, including physical touch. This type of early deprivation may undermine their ability to receive comfort from emotional relationships or form meaningful attachments for a lifetime.

While physical touch and other forms of TLC would likely benefit any traumatized child regardless of which behavioral changes they are exhibiting, those who are showing increased emotionality will likely be most receptive to this type of physical support. It might also feel most natural for you to give a soft back rub to a crying child as opposed to a kid who is withdrawing to his room or acting out by trashing the kitchen.

As a caveat, you also want your child to be comfortable turning away physical touch. The way I frame it for my patients is that children should be the boss of their own bodies. If you offer a hug and your child turns you down, it is crucial that you respect that boundary. This is, of course, true for any child, but especially so with a traumatized child whose trauma involved physical touch in some way (such as physical or sexual abuse).

When the trauma exposure involves touch, an unexpected pat on the back could morph into a trauma trigger. For this reason, if you see your little one crying or sucking her thumb and sense she could use a hug, ask permission before pulling her into a tight embrace and pay attention to how she responds to your touch after the fact.

Extra Attention

In addition to encouraging emotional expression, practicing validation, and using physical touch to communicate support, the skills
described in Chapter 3 can also benefit a traumatized child who is
increasingly emotional or is regressing developmentally. While physical touch is one way to communicate support, quality time is just as
important. Whether your son is suddenly speaking in a "babyish"
voice or your daughter is asking you to carry her up the stairs like you
did when she was a baby, these are signs your children would benefit
from quality time with their most trusted adult. Baking cookies, reading books, or getting on the floor for some play time could be the extra
attention they need.

Remember also to work in praise as appropriate. We will revisit
praise in the next chapter as it plays a crucial role in curbing minor
misbehavior, but for now, recall that praise can boost self-esteem and
increase behaviors you want to see more of, making the parent–child
relationship even more pleasant. Also recall that specific praise ("Nice
work cleaning up your blocks!" or "Thank you for sharing your art kit
with your sister") works better than general praise ("Atta boy!").

Active listening (also called *reflections*, covered in Chapter 3) can
be another effective way to help your child feel attended to. When
your child shares something with you—be it a feeling or something
that happened during the day—summarize it and repeat it back to the
child in your own words. For example, if your child shares having been
freaked out by a pop quiz in math class, you might say, "You were feeling really caught off guard when Ms. Smith sprung that quiz on you,
huh?" To add in some validation you might also say, "I hear ya. I used
to get so nervous during surprise exams too."

At the same time, we need to be specific and intentional in how
we dole out our extra attention. Because the function of the behavioral change (such as thumb sucking) is to garner more parental support, if you give your child extra attention and support, the behavior
is more likely to occur again. While this is good and normal when a

child is having some extra tears, be careful of how you respond if the regression involves toilet accidents or throwing tantrums.

Duane, a seven-year-old boy, started wetting the bed at night following his experience in a destructive hurricane. His father, wanting to give Duane lots of extra support and nurturance, would lovingly come into Duane's room each night when Duane called out to him, scoop him up, and carry him to the bathroom, singing to him softly as he changed Duane's clothes and bedsheets, and lying down for a few minutes with Duane in his clean bed. Sounds nice, right? Duane adores this middle-of-the-night special time with his father and, especially following his trauma, will not want to give it up. His father's heart is in the right place, but instead I would advise giving less attention to this type of behavior.*

Of course, your child will need fresh clothes and new bedsheets, but be careful not to turn this into a routine your child may cherish. It may help to keep in mind that assisting your little one with cleaning up the accident should be "all business" and then back to bed. This regression, like others, is still your child calling out for extra support, and they *should* get it—just not in the middle of the night after wetting the bed. Remember, parental attention makes any behavior more likely to occur. Duane's dad might consider carving out some special Duane–Dad time every evening before bed. If Duane is really into a Harry Potter phase, they could build this into the bedtime routine: Instead of walking Duane upstairs, tucking him in, and giving him a quick kiss good night, Dad could spend ten minutes cuddled up in bed with Duane while reading the latest chapter to him. This will give Duane a nice dose of physical touch and quality time, netting him the extra support he needs and deserves.

---

*There are a number of factors—other than trauma—that can cause bedwetting, including genetic influences and urinary tract infections. For this reason, bedwetting should always be evaluated by your child's pediatrician. Once your child's pediatrician has ruled out any medical issues or hormonal causes, and if the pediatrician has determined the bedwetting is voluntary—meaning your child wakes up before wetting the bed—you can treat bedwetting like any other regressive behavior.

The same principle of using parental attention to shape child behavior applies to minor misbehavior, which will be covered in the next chapter.

Each of these skills will help you navigate increased emotionality in your child. The take-home message is that increased emotionality and developmental regression are normal in a traumatized child. Furthermore, of all the behavioral changes a traumatized child might exhibit, these ones are relatively healthy, second only to a child using words to express feelings. Keep in mind that an over-the-top reaction to your child's tears or regression will only make it worse. Regressive behaviors can become more entrenched. Buried emotions will come out in other, more concerning ways. But by using active listening, validation, quality time, praise, and physical touch, you can support your child through a challenge that even the toughest adults can struggle with.

7

How to Respond to Minor Misbehavior

One evening after a family night out at the movies, Julian and his parents were shocked to find that someone had broken into their home. While there wasn't much damage and the stolen laptops could be replaced, Julian was still acting differently a month later. Instead of getting ready for school in the mornings, he has developed a habit of staying in bed playing video games. As a result he has missed his bus to elementary school several times. Having to drive Julian to school throws his mother off for the rest of the day. Yesterday, she was reprimanded at work for being late. This morning, she woke Julian up half an hour early to ensure he would be on time for his bus. When she called out to him, "Julian, you better not be playing that game" several times during the morning rush, each time he assured her he was getting ready. However, when 6:30 rolled around and Julian had still not made it downstairs, she went to check on him and found him in bed with his video game. His mother felt furious that he had lied and was going to make her late to work again. She immediately began yelling at him, called him "lazy" and "liar" and started trying to drag him out of bed. Julian then melted down into a tantrum that woke the rest of the house. Eventually, Julian made it downstairs and grabbed a breakfast bar for the car, and his mother sped him to school. She was late to work again.

What happened here?

A therapist might call Julian's initial behavior noncompliance. This is one of many behaviors that can be classified as minor misbehavior. Repeatedly ignoring a parent's request to clean up a room, using "bad words" or swearing, and whining or throwing a temper tantrum when they don't get their way are some of the most common ways we see children misbehave. While children of all ages and backgrounds typically exhibit some of these behaviors over the course of their childhood, these behaviors may increase in frequency or intensity following a trauma.

The simplest explanation for why traumatized children might act out more is that they are having a hard time.

As we saw in Chapters 4 and 6, trauma can be like trying to hold an inflated beach ball under the water in a pool. After a traumatic experience, your child may want to push down painful thoughts, feelings, and trauma-related memories. But like keeping down the beach ball, it's hard work pushing down these thoughts and feelings—hard work that is essentially impossible to sustain. Like the beach ball, these suppressed thoughts and feelings may come erupting out of the water at any time in a number of different ways, including misbehavior.

For decades, therapists have encouraged frustrated parents to reframe their aggravated thoughts about these eruptions: Your kids are not giving you a hard time; they're *having* a hard time.

At the same time, Julian's mom still needs to get to work on time and he needs to get to school.

If you've made it this far in the book, you probably have the sense that yelling at your son is not likely to make things better. But it's important to understand why parental responses like yelling aren't effective.

Not only is it unkind to yell at your child—which threatens to inflict serious damage on your relationship—it also just doesn't work. Strong feelings impede learning, and there are few feelings stronger than fear. When Julian's mom stormed into his room with a raised voice, hurling insults, he undoubtedly had some strong feelings about it. This is true for any child, but especially for children following a traumatic event. The fight–flight–freeze response is already primed, and kids are ready to overreact to any perceived threat. This applies to a potentially traumatic experience—like when Julian's home was burglarized—as well as something more commonplace, like his mother's yelling.

Research also supports the idea that stress and fear impair learning: Several studies have demonstrated that children experiencing stress and fear score significantly lower on IQ tests than their stress-free counterparts. The neurological basis for this was covered in Chapter 4: When a child is feeling scared or stressed out, the child's amygdala becomes activated, kicking off a stress response that involves the entire body. When this happens, activation in the prefrontal cortex is decreased, and thinking, learning, and decision-making abilities all become impaired.

To put it simply: Being stressed out makes it hard to learn.

So what does this mean for Julian and his noncompliance? It means insults and raised voices likely will not curb his noncompliance. Instead, his needs for extra support and attention will go unmet. He will be left feeling stressed, thinking that his mom doesn't like him, and turn to his video game to detach from it all.

Clearly Julian's mom needs a different tactic if she wants her son to change his behavior.

Selective Attention and Praise

As we discussed in Chapter 6, parental attention is the single strongest force that can shape a child's behavior. With that in mind, the first skill introduced for responding to minor misbehavior is called *selective attention*. Since fear-based punishment is often ineffective, and parental attention is the strongest shaper of child behavior, selective attention posits that a behavior that is met with parental attention will increase and a behavior ignored by parents will decrease.

That should seem pretty obvious, but here's the tricky part that many parents don't understand at first: It doesn't matter if the attention is positive or negative! Chiding a daughter for coloring on the walls and praising a son for drawing a beautiful picture on a piece of construction paper may both reward a child's behavior with parental attention.

Parents who yell at children displaying minor misbehavior might inadvertently be reinforcing them to act out *more*. Kids are not going to understand and learn whatever the yelling parent is trying to communicate—remember, it is hard to learn while stressed. And on an unconscious level, they'll be more likely to engage in the behavior again, especially if their needs for attention and control are not otherwise being met.

Consider the following example:

Sadie is a seven-year-old girl who lives with her grandmother and was traumatized after her house burned down. Like any child, she would occasionally whine or throw a temper tantrum before her trauma exposure. But in the months following the fire, her tantrums have picked up in both frequency and intensity. It has gotten to the point where her grandmother is afraid to take Sadie out in public. Sadie's grandmother is a sensitive, thoughtful woman, and this is evident in the way she responds to Sadie's tantrums. Knowing that they've picked up in part due to Sadie's home burning down, her grandmother tries to comfort, console, and appease her every time Sadie melts down. While waiting for a therapy session one day, Sadie sees a chocolate bar in the waiting room vending machine. She wants it badly, and when her grandmother initially turns her down, reminding her that it's nearly dinnertime, Sadie starts crying and yelling, "I want it now!" Her grandmother rubs her back and gently tries to set a boundary around dinnertime, but Sadie forges ahead, yelling louder and louder until her grandmother gives in and buys her the chocolate bar.

Sadie has learned two very important things in this situation:

1. Throwing a tantrum will get her attention from grandmother.

2. If she simply cries loud enough and long enough, she will probably get what she wants.

Sadie's grandmother learned something too: If she gives Sadie what she wants, the tantrum will stop. Parents may think they're in charge of the relationship, but just as much as we train our children, they train us too.

What could Sadie's grandmother do differently?

I like to say that using selective attention actually starts when your child is behaving well. Selective attention only works if there is a stark contrast to the ignoring.

Here's how to do it: When your child is behaving well, give the child a lot of attention. If the child is doing something that delights you (like sharing a toy with a sibling), make sure you praise him for it!

Flip back to Chapter 3 for detailed instructions on how to dole out specific praise. The basic rule is to specifically label the behavior you want to see more of instead of something more general (for example, "Thank you for sharing your crayons with your little brother; you're a great big sister" versus "Nice job!").

Something else I might add is that while specific praise given to your child is important, feel free to sing the child's praises to others too. Sadie might really respond to overhearing her grandmother brag to her grandfather about how well she listened to her after their therapy appointment.

But not every behavior is praiseworthy. Some are neutral, and it might feel phony to try to praise something like that ("You're doing so great playing with that toy!").

With younger children, you can attend to your child's more neutral behaviors by simply noticing and acknowledging them. Parent–child interaction therapy (PCIT) is an evidence-based therapy approach often applied to teach parents how to respond to misbehaving traumatized children; it refers to this skill as *giving descriptions*. A helpful way the developers of this model frame it is to think of yourself as a sportscaster narrating what your child is doing—be the Bob Costas to your own personal dream team. Think: "Oh, I see you're reading *The Very Hungry Caterpillar*" or "Now you're drawing a picture of a giraffe." Again, when your children feel like you're paying attention to them—whether positive, negative, or neutral—their behavior is reinforced. For more information on PCIT, turn to Chapter 11.

By praising them for behaviors you'd like to see more of *and* noticing and acknowledging their neutral behaviors, you will be giving your children a lot of attention. This ensures that their need for attention is more likely to be met, and it serves up a stark contrast when you withdraw that attention. Even during the best times, this practice of selective attention and praise can help your child be happy, be productive, and avoid tantrums. When your child is stressed after a trauma, it can help get the child back on the right track.

Reflecting and Validating

Beyond laying the groundwork for reinforcement through praise, you can offer up a quick bit of comfort by guessing at what your child might be feeling (see Chapters 3 and 6 for information on active listening and validation). For Sadie's grandmother, this may sound like "You're feeling really frustrated because you want that candy bar, huh?" Sometimes, a little bit of understanding may be all you need to disarm a tantrum. In these cases, all the child needed was to feel heard, understood, and acknowledged. I also encourage caregivers to offer up a statement like this because it gives a name to the emotion the child may be experiencing, increasing emotional literacy. This is especially important for young children, who often lack the vocabulary to express their thoughts and feelings.

Ignoring

However, often a bit of comfort and understanding is not enough. What comes next?

My answer stems from a simple but radical premise: Ignore it.

Instead of yelling like Julian's mom or giving in like Sadie's grandmother, turn your attention away and keep it away as long as your child is engaging in the behavior. As soon as your child does something that is not whining for the candy bar—provided it's not more misbehavior—attend to the behavior immediately, with either praise or sportscasting. Here's what it might look like with Sadie and her grandmother, mid-tantrum, after Grandma has already offered some support:

SADIE: Ahhhh! I don't care about stupid dinner! I need that candy!

GRANDMOTHER: (*turns away from Sadie, takes a seat on a chair next to the vending machine, picks up a* Highlights *magazine about sharks*)

SADIE: You have to get it for me NOW!

GRANDMOTHER: (*keeps a calm look on her face, continues flipping through the magazine*)

SADIE: Now, now, now!

GRANDMOTHER: (*continues flipping through magazine*)

SADIE: Ahhhhhhh!

GRANDMOTHER: Ah, a feature on Great Whites (*to herself, while looking down at the magazine*).

SADIE: (*whines*)

GRANDMOTHER: (*keeps flipping through magazine*)*

SADIE: (*takes a few steps over to Grandma, peers at the magazine*)

---

*It's normal for this process of planned ignoring to take several minutes, though it can feel like a lot longer. Expect for it to take the longest for your child to "get it" the first few times you implement selective attention.

GRANDMOTHER: Ooh, you're checking out that big mouth of teeth.

SADIE: One time my friend Janie's uncle found one of the teeth on the beach. She said it was kinda small.

GRANDMOTHER: Wow, that's really neat! Thank you for coming over to tell me about that.

Having to stand up to your kids like this is no fun for anyone. It is a bit like being a hostage negotiator in a blockbuster action movie: We don't negotiate with terrorists. But you don't want to be some tough guy in these situations. After all, you're still a loving parent. Sometimes I like to think of how former secretary of state James Baker once described diplomacy: like being an iron fist in a velvet glove. You should be kind and gentle, but unyielding in your stance.

Beware the Extinction Burst

An extinction burst is an increase in an undesirable behavior that can happen when you first start to implement selective attention or ignoring. If you've given in to your child's whines and tantrums like Sadie's grandmother has, your child might whine louder or tantrum longer in a bid to get that attention they're used to getting from misbehavior. Hold the course. It might feel overwhelming or embarrassing in the moment, but know you're doing the right thing and that eventually your child will get the message, and the behavior will be extinguished.

While selective attention is typically the first intervention I prescribe for parenting traumatized children with behavior issues, it can seem a little cruel to ignore them for behaving in a way that they don't know is wrong. For this reason, I encourage parents to pair selective attention with explicitly setting and holding boundaries.

Setting and Holding Boundaries

Setting boundaries and enforcing consequences is something that many parents struggle with. We can all understand why Julian's mom feels frazzled in the mornings, especially after getting reprimanded at work, and we can also understand why some parents might feel tempted to yell in stressful situations. At the same time, we can also probably empathize with a caregiver who is overly permissive with their traumatized child, like Sadie's grandmother, fearing the child might be too fragile for discipline. After what you have read in Chapters 1–6, you know your children might be scared, hurting, and confused, and you know that acting-out behaviors are likely just a way for them to protect themselves. You also know your crucial role in helping them heal. With all of that in mind, giving them anything other than skillful support and good old-fashioned TLC can feel wrong.

But there's also something about setting boundaries and enforcing consequences that can help a child—especially a traumatized one—feel safe.

The rationale behind this stems from something else you've already learned: Children commonly feel out of control after experiencing something terrifying. To go back to Chapter 1, a traumatic experience can shatter a child's assumptions about the world. While they once felt safe, now they fear something bad may happen every time they leave the home. When a parent sets consistent rules that a child can count on, and enforces boundaries when those rules are broken, the family becomes a place where the child feels safe and contained. When parents let their traumatized child have ice cream for lunch when there had been a prior rule about having balanced meals, or suddenly tells their traumatized child they don't actually need to share their toys anymore, their world is further thrown into chaos. Which way is up?

Aside from the benefits of consistency, it also communicates to your child that you are the leader of your family. In times of tumult, it can be comforting to know that someone else—someone more mature who has the child's best interests in mind—is calling the shots.

But how do you set and hold a boundary?

* *Frame it positively:* Telling your child "Don't do this" or "No, not like that" is more likely to inspire pushback and resentment than framing it as a positive. Think back to Julian and his mom. Instead of saying, "Julian, you better not be playing that game," she could try "Julian, time to get out of bed."

* *Be specific:* Again, instead of making a comment about his game, Julian's mom could issue a more specific directive ("It's time to come to the kitchen for breakfast").

* *Provide a rationale:* You will get more "buy-in" from your child if you provide a brief, simple explanation of the boundary, especially if it's a new rule. The goal here is not to overwhelm your child with a long explanation, but if you're introducing something new to a routine, it will help to explain why you're issuing the additional directive (for example, "It's important to be on time for school so that I can get to work on time").

* *Hold the line:* If your child tries to ignore the boundary, you have a few options. With younger children, it's easier to be more hands on. If Julian is a young child, his mother might consider going into his room and physically helping him get out of bed and get dressed. The consequence for young Julian's misbehavior is that he lost some autonomy in the ability to get up and get himself dressed. This obviously wouldn't work with an older child. If Julian were a teen, the more appropriate way to hold the line would be to enforce a different consequence, such as removing access to his video game.

To see selective attention and boundary setting in action, consider the case of seven-year-old Jackie, who was traumatized after being attacked by the neighbor's dogs:

DAD: All right, kids, who is ready for pizza for dinner?

JACKIE: Yuck, your pizza is gross.

DAD: We sit together as a family at dinnertime, and it's important we fill up our stomachs at dinner so we don't get hungry at night. You are welcome to make something else for yourself if you like.

JACKIE: Eew. I'm not eating that.

DAD: (*turns to sibling*) So, Jeremy, how was school today?

JACKIE: (*rolls eyes*)

DAD: (*eats his own meal, continues attending to brother*)

JACKIE: This is so gross.

DAD: (*continues to ignore Jackie*)

JACKIE: (*stands up and makes herself a peanut butter and jelly sandwich*)

DAD: Nice job making your own dinner, Jackie.

In this example, Jackie's dad ignores her insults about his pizza, sets a boundary around dinnertime (we sit together as a family), and provides a rationale for why it's important to eat dinner (to fill our stomachs up so we don't get hungry in the night). This isn't enough to curb Jackie's sassiness, so her father moves into selective attention and ignores her behavior. As soon as she stands up to make something else for herself, she earns praise from Dad.

Keep in mind that these tactics are also effective in responding to minor misbehavior in children who haven't experienced adverse events. With traumatized children, however, it's even more important to stay consistent with these practices so that your behavior and limits are predictable to your child. This predictability lends itself to a sense of safety, which is crucial for traumatized children. Additionally, this practice will help curb the minor misbehaviors that sometimes increase with trauma.

Most frequently, when a child exhibits minor misbehavior following a trauma, it is a sign that the child is struggling internally and needs a little extra attention from you. But whether it's an attempt to boss you around ("You can't sit next to me!"), yelling at you for no apparent reason ("I hate you!"), or demanding special privileges ("You need to buy me these three Xbox games right now!"), these behaviors can get aggravating and get in the way of your family's everyday life. By using your attention to shape your child's behavior you will be able to meet the child's increased needs for support and decrease the acting out. But sometimes you can use these skills all you want, and your child may still buck or even escalate. At times, misbehavior can transform from simply annoying to absolutely not okay (for example, physical aggression, destruction of property). If this is the case for your family, see Chapter 9, where we will discuss how to respond to major misbehavior.

8

Handling Withdrawal and Avoidance

As discussed in Chapter 1, some kids develop posttraumatic stress disorder (PTSD) after experiencing something scary, while others encountering the exact same stressor do not. One major factor that can make the difference is whether the child tries to avoid reminders of the scary incident.

It's perfectly normal for our children to try to forget about their trauma. After all, any reminders can bring back uncomfortable thoughts and upsetting feelings. However, the act of turning away from trauma reminders for the sake of immediate relief sets off a vicious cycle in which these nonthreatening situations can make children's long-term anxiety worse and keep them prisoner in their own mind. Something as ubiquitous as the sound of an ambulance can become a terrifying trigger. Something as idiosyncratic as a man who has the same type of facial hair as the perpetrator of an assault can cause a flurry of painful emotions.

Gabriel was thrilled to get his driver's license on his sixteenth birthday. One of his favorite things afforded by his new freedom was the ability to drive to the coffee shop on the way to school and meet up with his friends on Friday mornings. On one such morning, his car is T-boned in a hit-and-run. Terrified, shaken, and all alone, Gabriel sits frozen at the wheel for several minutes, unsure of what to do. Eventually a police officer drives by and comes to Gabriel's aid. The car is totaled, and Gabriel is left feeling shocked, sore, and afraid. Months later, after insurance claims have been sorted and Gabriel is physically healed, he still refuses to drive. He asks his mother to drive him to school but turns down her offer to drop him off at the coffee shop on Friday mornings. She wants Gabriel to drive again and connect with his friends. However, seeing the look of fear on her son's face is all it takes for her to agree to follow his lead. Gabriel starts exhibiting some symptoms of depression in addition to all this fear—he seems down all the time and is typically isolated in his room all weekend long. Eventually, he stops talking to his friends altogether. While he used to beg his mom to let him keep his phone at his bedside overnight so he could respond to any texts that came through, he now leaves his phone around the house, not bothering to check for messages. His mom can't remember the last time he connected with his friends at all.

It makes perfect sense that Gabriel wants to avoid getting behind the wheel. In his mind, driving himself has become unsafe, and reminders of the accident, like the coffee shop, bring back some of the upsetting feelings he felt the day of the hit-and-run. This type of avoidance is powerful: By enlisting his mom to do the driving, Gabriel can temporarily decrease his anxiety and feel like he's keeping himself safe. What's so wrong with that?

Unfortunately, this type of avoidance is not as innocuous as it may seem. First, his anxieties about driving begin to snowball. The more he avoids it, the scarier it gets. But it's not just his increasing anxiety—it's about how this fear can shrink Gabriel's world. Instead of enjoying his weekly coffee with friends and newfound freedom, he's being driven to school by his mom. This dynamic—avoiding age-appropriate behavior—may cause him to feel some shame. It's understandable that a teenager in this situation might begin to feel depressed and resign himself to long weekends shuttered away in his bedroom, where he feels safe—if sad.

Before we jump into how Gabriel's mom might offer an effective response, let's think about all the factors that could be contributing to Gabriel's avoidance.

• *Obvious triggers:* We can all understand why a kid like Gabriel might be afraid to get behind the wheel again—it feels unsafe to him. It also makes sense that this fear would make him want to avoid driving and going to the coffee shop.

• *Less obvious triggers:* Gabriel might also feel fear when he sees his friends peel out of the coffee shop parking lot or when they ask him if he wants a ride to school. His friends and parents might not notice the beads of sweat that build on his brow whenever Gabriel is reminded of the reckless driver who smashed into his car.

• *Decreased energy:* Feelings of exhaustion are common in posttraumatic stress. This could be caused by sleep impairment, a common symptom of posttraumatic stress, the psychological toll of having the fight–flight–freeze response triggered so frequently, or by depression, which can grow in tandem with avoidance.

• *Loss of interest:* In some children, loss of interest or pleasure in their usual activities—another symptom typically associated with depression—can emerge after they've been traumatized. Anxiety can also fuel withdrawal from typical hobbies and pursuits. Gabriel's fears, for example, compel him to stop hanging out with his friends.

• *Shame:* Gabriel may harbor some feelings of embarrassment or shame about the accident—and also about his fear arising from the accident. He might be having inaccurate or unhelpful negative thoughts like "What kind of loser is afraid to get in the car with a friend?" or "I'll never be normal again." Beating themselves up and making unrealistic predictions can cause traumatized children and adolescents to withdraw further.

• *Insensitivity from others:* It's not just about Gabriel's internalized sense of shame. He also might be getting feedback from his friends or family that is insensitive and makes him want to withdraw. In my practice, I've heard from countless patients whose well-meaning friends or siblings make a friendly jab after a visible startle response or newfound fear.

So what are Gabriel and his mom to do?

Exposure

The answer to the problem of avoidance is a straightforward yet counterintuitive one: exposure. Instead of avoiding trauma reminders that bring about anxiety, people need to approach them. This is often easier said than done when you have an anxious or traumatized child on your hands. Much of this book is focused on how to support your child, and guiding a child to do something that feels uncomfortable can seem counter to that message. However, I encourage you to think of exposure not as throwing your child to the wolves, but instead as walking up to a pack of big dogs, hand in hand, and helping your child realize these seemingly scary animals are actually fluffy playmates. Just think of how the kids from the film *The Sandlot* were so terrified of "the Beast" until they realized the baseball-devouring hound was actually a friendly neighborhood pet who just loved to chase balls. Scotty Smalls and the gang could have saved themselves a lot of trouble if they had just walked up to the friendly—if humongous—canine and said hello rather than let their imaginations run wild.

Of course when you're dealing with a kid who may have a powerful imagination and strong emotions, it might not be as simple as that.

To understand how exposure works, consider the behavioral principle of *habituation*. Habituation refers to the diminishing physiological or psychological response to a frequently repeated situation. In our context, it means that your child will eventually get used to approaching the things she avoids if done again and again. Instead of creating a fear response, these once-scary things and places will become commonplace, even boring. Your child will become increasingly brave with each exposure. She will see her anxiety decreasing and realize the supposed terror she has been avoiding is actually not so dangerous at all. This of course only applies to situations that are not inherently dangerous. If, for example, the dog next door does sometimes attack children, exposure is not only unwise, but also unlikely to be effective.

Another important component of effective exposure is that it be done *gradually*. You aren't trying to throw your kid into the deep end of the pool without warning, but rather to help him stick his foot in a few times, followed by both legs, and slowly wade in before dunking his head under water. This means you can take your time and start by helping your child approach the trauma reminders that cause only a little bit of anxiety. Once the child has mastered that, he can approach reminders that cause a little more anxiety, followed eventually by those that cause the most anxiety. It's also important not to expect anxiety about trauma reminders to disappear instantly after the first exposure. It can take time.

Consider this example of a parent supporting a child after a scary bike accident:

Olivia was riding her bike around her neighborhood when she hit a pothole and flew off her bike, scraping her knees and hands and bruising her chin. Even after her injuries healed, Olivia sadly insisted her bike riding days were over. Rather than accept this proclamation, her father helped her come up with a plan to conquer her fears. They lowered the seat on her bike so that her feet could easily touch the ground at any moment, and her dad accompanied her on a quick ride down their street. Olivia felt a little nervous about this but had a good time laughing with her dad, joking around about her riding her "clown bike" around the street. Once she felt totally comfortable with this, her father raised her bike seat a little more, where she could still reach the ground from her bike seat, but only on her tiptoes. Because it was only a little higher, Olivia only felt a bit nervous. They rode down the street together again, until it became boring to Olivia. Olivia and her dad moved forward like this until one day she felt brave enough to ride around her block by herself with her bike seat at the proper position.

We will go into the steps involved in preparing for and carrying out an exposure later in the chapter, but for now keep in mind that Olivia's dad harnessing his close, jovial relationship with his daughter was just as important as the exposure itself.

Before You Start: Is Therapy Necessary?

With a kid like Gabriel, a car accident could result in mild anxiety and avoidance that can be addressed similarly to how Olivia's dad helped her get over her fear of bike riding. His mom could accompany him on a few drives around the block, encourage him to accept a ride from a friend, and ultimately work up to driving himself to school again. On the other hand, if a kid like Gabriel is experiencing terror at the prospect of driving, fear of this intensity is better addressed with the support of a therapist.

It may seem hard to make a call on exactly how distressed your child is.

Consider using the Subjective Units of Distress Scale (SUDS), originally developed by Dr. Joseph Wolpe in his 1969 book, *The Practice of Behavior Therapy*, as a way to gauge your child's anxiety. It's a quick and easy way to help you sort out the intensity of your child's experience that has been in use for more than fifty years in various forms, with descriptors for the scale ratings adjusted to fit each clinician's purposes. In therapy, this type of scale might be used to help craft a list of exposure targets or to help organize the order of potential exposures from mild to moderate to intense.

I typically present this to patients by asking "On a zero to ten scale, if zero is the best you could possibly feel and ten is the worst, where would you rate yourself right now?" See the box on the next page for more detail on the scale.

The SUDS Scale for Gauging Anxiety

0: At complete peace, no worries whatsoever.

1: Feeling great, only minimal anxiety that you would have to focus on to notice.

2: Still feeling pretty good; some worries, but they are more annoying than anything.

3: Mildly anxious; you can ignore it with some effort.

4: Somewhat anxious; you can't easily ignore it.

5: Moderately anxious; hard to distract yourself from it.

6: Increasingly anxious; it's impossible to ignore.

7: Starting to panic, but you can maintain control with a lot of effort.

8: Very anxious, struggling to control your emotions.

9: Feeling desperately anxious, starting to lose control of your emotions.

10: Any control over emotions is long gone; feeling absolutely terrible.

If your child feels mildly anxious (say, less than 5) and open to the idea of approaching something he would rather avoid, and you feel comfortable supporting him in it (that is, you're willing to ride around the block in the passenger seat ten times), go for it. If instead your child's distress seems moderate to intense and he is disturbed by this idea, therapy is the better choice.

Other factors to consider:

• What type of adverse event did your child experience? Trauma caused by commonplace single-incident events like a car crash, bike accident, or a dog bite that didn't require any medical intervention can respond well to some parent-supported exposure. Children traumatized by more complex, ongoing events like sexual abuse, bullying, or repeated community violence are often better supported by a therapist.

- Does the avoided situation seem safe to you? Eating at restaurants, riding bikes, driving cars, and meeting friends at coffee shops are often relatively harmless activities. If you aren't sure if your child's situation is safe, consult a therapist.

- Is your child traumatized, or does she just have some residual anxiety? Think back to Chapter 2. If you've determined your child has been traumatized and has ongoing symptoms of posttraumatic stress (say, over one month after the event) that interfere with everyday life, you should seek professional help. In this case, exposure is best tackled with a therapist. If your child doesn't exhibit any posttraumatic stress symptoms beyond some mild avoidance, and this avoidance doesn't impact things like her performance in school or relationships with friends and family, therapy might not be necessary.

Consider the case of a seven-year-old boy who witnessed a robbery while enjoying a Happy Meal at McDonald's. He was shaken up after the incident, but as far as his parents can tell, he's doing well in school, remains close to his friends, and is still his affable self at home with family. He seems to be eating, sleeping, and playing much the same way he was before experiencing this adverse event. The only thing his parents notice is he refuses to eat out at any fast-food restaurants. He feels bummed about his fears, because he can't join his friends at McDonald's for an upcoming birthday party. He recently remarked to his mother, "I wish I could go to that party." This boy would be an ideal candidate for parent-assisted exposure: He has very few posttraumatic stress symptoms, a single-incident trauma, and he is motivated to overcome a fear of an innocuous situation. Some other examples might be a girl who had her purse stolen in a parking lot and became apprehensive and avoidant of all parking lots but is otherwise her normal self. Or a boy who stopped attending the camping trips he used to love after one outdoor trek was ruined by a freak weather event that he's convinced put his life in danger.

Preparing For and Carrying Out Exposure

With the boy who is sad to be missing out on the McDonald's birthday celebration, his mom could follow these steps:

1. **Share an example of what exposure looks like:** His mom could share something like the story on pages 134–135 about Olivia falling off her bike, being afraid to ride again, and getting support from her father.

2. **Gauge whether a similar plan would be appropriate for your child:** If her son seems interested in the example, his anxiety is minimal, and he doesn't have much in the way of posttraumatic stress symptoms, his mother could say, "Is this something you'd like to try with me?"

3. **Collaborate on an exposure plan:** Identify small steps that could lead up to attending the party. For our mother–son pair working on the fear of McDonald's, these could include visiting different fast-food restaurants (for example, Burger King, Wendy's), going through the McDonald's drive-through, visiting different McDonald's locations, and finally, visiting the McDonald's where the robbery occurred.

4. **Move through the plan:** Once he habituates to a step (that is, it stops eliciting a fear response), it's time to move to the next step until the boy gets used to the McDonald's he's most fearful of.

5. **Know when to stop:** If his fear ever increases to moderate or severe levels, it's time to call in a therapist. The therapist may want to pursue more parent-supported exposures, but in that case you can rely on the professional's judgment about when to challenge your child rather than forging ahead on your own. On the other hand, when your child has habituated to the fear and seems no longer afraid, this is a wonderful stopping point. In younger children, you may notice they start to get bored with the exposures. For teens, it sometimes manifests as annoyance. Not quite sure? Check in with your child. With the boy in the story above, his mom might simply ask if he feels ready to go to the party.

What If the Child Isn't Motivated?

I have seen plenty of children who, after being exposed to an adverse event, become comfortable in their avoidance. One of the most common examples of this is kids who relish sleeping with caregivers and avoid their own rooms. While this avoidance is a little more complex—it may have less to do with their specific trauma than with fears of being alone or in the dark—the way we treat it is the same. Start by introducing the concept of exposure, then break it down into little, manageable steps. This might look like having your child sleep in a sleeping bag on the floor instead of with you in the bed. This is an ideal first step because not only does it give your child time to habituate gradually, but it's not quite as comfortable as snuggling up to Mom or Dad on a comfortable mattress with eight-hundred-thread-count bedsheets—and it can make your child's own bed seem appealing by comparison. After this, you could step down to lying down with your child until the child falls asleep in her own bedroom.

If your child fights against the exposure process, whether because he simply doesn't want to change habits or is earnestly afraid, here is my advice: Don't push it. This is when it's time to involve a therapist.

Of course, your child will eventually need to sleep in his own room again, but this is not something you want to cause a power struggle over, especially for a traumatized child. Our primary goal is for you to stay in the position of number-one supporter, and getting into a tense fight about something that makes him feel uncomfortable can quickly derail that.

What Parent-Assisted Exposure Might Look Like in a Variety of Situations

Still confused about whether or not your child might be an appropriate candidate for parent-assisted exposure or what this exposure might look like? First, remember that these two criteria must be met for parent-assisted exposure:

1. Your child should be functioning about as well as ever in different aspects of life outside of the avoidance that is causing problems.

2. The child should be open or curious about trying exposure with you.

Here are some examples of how exposure might unfold:

Incident: An eight-year-old girl breaks her wrist playing capture the flag in PE class, and now she not only refuses to take part in gym class at school but also is asking her parents to let her drop out of her soccer league, despite her love for the sport.

Exposure: If the child is unable to take part in physical activities, the parent can start by simply watching sports with the girl from the sidelines. Once cleared by her physician, Mom or Dad could try some gentle one-on-one games of catch or passing the soccer ball back and forth. Then bring in siblings or friends for a casual scrimmage. Eventually, work back up to participating in PE class and taking part in team sports.

Incident: A ten-year-old boy was walking his corgi when a neighbor's territorial chow chow got off-leash and attacked the boy's dog. He's now afraid to take his pet anywhere, despite his neighbor's rehoming the aggressive canine.

Exposure: The parent can accompany the child on outings with their corgi, including walks, visits to the groomer, or trips to the dog park, starting with whichever causes him the least anxiety and working up to what is most stressful.

Incident: A sixteen-year-old girl got serious food poisoning after eating out at a restaurant and now begs her family to stop their Sunday night tradition of eating out.

Exposure: The parents can start by having their daughter accompany them to a restaurant while they eat, working up to her ordering small portions or foods that seem more "safe" (for example, buttered noodles).

When Your Child Is Avoiding You

While avoidance can drive a child straight into her parents' bedroom, avoidance can also drive a wedge between children and their caregivers. Sometimes this is because caregivers can serve as trauma reminders. Picture a child whose sexual assault was stopped by her mother, or a child who was staying with his grandfather when he had a stroke. This avoidance is fairly straightforward. The person the child avoids is directly tied to the child's adverse experience. At the same time, kids with posttraumatic stress may avoid their friends, family, and activities for reasons other than their tie to a trauma.

After her romantic relationship with a popular boy ended, Jeri found herself on the receiving end of some nasty school bullying. It culminated in Jeri's getting slapped by one of her ex-boyfriend's female friends during lunchtime in the school cafeteria. The school responded appropriately by separating the girls before the fight could escalate and suspending Jeri's bully. Jeri never showed any of the classic avoidance symptoms—she still eats lunch in the cafeteria every day. But for some reason she refuses to come down to the dinner table with her family. Jeri's parents are spinning their wheels trying to help her. She feels exhausted by her mom's nagging attempts to "talk about it," or her dad's pointing out what she could do differently the next time she's approached by a bully so that she could "win." The worst part for Jeri is that her parents have made it clear they are trying to get her bully expelled—she felt humiliated when she saw her mother coming out of the principal's office days after the incident. Jeri would rather keep her head down and go about business as usual.

What's going on here?

- This poor girl has dealt with enough already. Bullying can overwhelm anyone, and Jeri's parents, though their hearts are in the right place, may be adding to her level of stress. This stress prompts her to shut down, withdraw, and avoid.

- Jeri may have some shame about getting slapped. Her dad's focus on "winning" a fight may be inadvertently sending the message that Jeri was a "loser" for being hit. And the obvious attempts at getting the bully kicked out of school only double down on the message that Jeri can't take care of herself.

If your child doesn't want to talk with you about being bullied, that's not necessarily a function of trauma or pathological avoidance. Jeri may be completely fine, if a little embarrassed or ashamed. Her biggest stressors may be her parents' invasive attempts at supporting her, and she may be one of the majority of kids who go on to heal naturally after experiencing a potentially traumatic event. If this is the case, her avoidance of her parents is not only normal, but a way of protecting herself. If your child says she is fine, and avoidance is only showing up at home, it could be worthwhile to reflect on how you might be contributing to your child's behavior instead of assuming something is wrong with your child.

If you're spinning your wheels over this and can't seem to figure out whether your child is suffering from posttraumatic avoidance or is simply wanting some space from you, flip back to Chapter 2 for guidance on how to determine if your child has been traumatized. Still confused? You might consider consulting a therapist for yourself. We will cover this more in Chapter 11. But for now just keep in mind that any parent can feel overwhelmed after learning their child has experienced something terrifying, and there is no shame in seeking some support to cope with this. Anyone can understand Jeri's parents' desperation to support their daughter and get her bully kicked out of school—they want to protect their child. At the same time, her parents could benefit from getting some perspective on how Jeri might feel about it all.

Finally, there are some circumstances when avoidance is truly the healthiest response. If the triggering event that caused the underlying trauma was truly dangerous, then it may make sense to let your child stay away. I once saw a patient who loved climbing precariously high on a neighborhood oak tree, much to his parents' worry. One day after a rainstorm he tried to climb to his usual height, lost his grip on the slippery bark, and broke both arms. His parents were terrified after hearing a thud and scream—but also relieved it wasn't worse. When their son decided he didn't want to climb trees anymore, the parents were more than happy to let him stick to the well-padded jungle gym at the local playground.

To wrap things up: While Jeri's parents responded to her avoidance with alarm, other parents may overlook avoidance symptoms, especially in contrast to the other behavior changes we may see after trauma. After all, your child isn't crying, misbehaving, hurting himself, or otherwise acting in a way that calls for your immediate attention. Addressing avoidance may seem less pressing than other, more shocking trauma symptoms. However, we know that these insidious symptoms can be some of the most worrisome because of how they can snowball and limit your child's world. This can lead to isolation and, ultimately, feelings of depression, as they did with Gabriel, who avoided driving following his car accident. That is why it is so important to make sure you're getting the support necessary to help your child heal. Don't be afraid to seek out a therapist if exposure attempts are met with fear, opposition, or anxiety. But if your child seems interested and amenable to exposure, and his distress is mild, feel free to take the lead. With a caring, informed parent who is oriented to exposure principles (and maybe therapeutic support too), your child can overcome the vicious cycle of avoidance and go on to live an empowered life.

9

Dealing with Major Misbehavior

There's a moment every parent knows is coming but is rarely prepared to handle: the moment your son first rolls his eyes at you. Or maybe it's when your sweet daughter starts sassing you and talking back. Or when they take to stomping off to their room, demanding they be left alone. Inevitably, your child is going to start growing up and begin changing into someone different from the little sweetheart who used to tug on your shirt and was desperate for your approval.

Even though the minor misbehavior and withdrawal behaviors addressed in Chapters 7 and 8 frequently increase after a trauma, many parents are quick to consider these behavioral changes a normal, but unfortunate, part of growing up. And sometimes they are. Other times, however, these changes can get a little more serious—and scary—than the symptoms we've addressed in past chapters. In my own practice, I rarely get calls from parents of a child worried about why she wants to skip the family vacation or has started acting rude. But I get plenty of panicked parents pleading for a same-day appointment the moment their child first starts exhibiting alarming acting-out behaviors.

Maybe their child trashed his room, crashed the family car, or started a fight at school. This is what therapists refer to as major misbehavior. Among younger kids, major misbehavior typically involves throwing toys, hitting and biting other kids or adults, and dangerous noncompliance—such as running into the street or trying to get away from parents in a busy mall. In older kids, major misbehavior can involve truly scary physical aggression, such as punching holes in walls at home or giving a classmate a black eye. It can also entail dangerously reckless behavior, such as getting in car crashes or abusing drugs and alcohol. (We'll cover the specifics of posttraumatic teenage impulsivity in more depth in Chapter 10.) In this chapter, we are going to review the different ways major misbehavior can manifest itself, how to make sense of this problem, and what you can do to help manage and reduce major acting-out episodes. Let's start with an example:

Campbell and Jaxon are nine-year-old twins who are obsessed with their PlayStation 5. Their parents have a hard time pulling the boys away for school, dinner, and bedtime. They wanted to have some boundaries around video game playtime, but they often let the boys play for hours on end because they're simply relieved to see their sons having a good time. Jaxon was recently traumatized after discovering a neighbor who had overdosed on drugs. In the following weeks, their once-gleeful boy had been sullen, oversleeping, and generally shut down. The appearance of a brand-new video game system has seemed to put an end to all of that negativity.

One day, their younger sister, Ashleigh, eager to join the boys in their fun, tries to serve them some fruit juice while they are playing. She trips over a cord and accidentally spills juice all over the gaming system. The boys are furious. They both yell at her and make her cry, but Jaxon goes further. He seemingly loses control, grabbing Ashleigh by her arms and yelling in her face, threatening to beat her up. Campbell restrains his brother, trying to get him to calm down, when Jaxon turns and takes a swing at him. Hearing the commotion, their mom comes into the room, scoops up Ashleigh, and then desperately tries to calm Jaxon down by promising to buy him a new PlayStation 5. Later that night she relates the scene to her husband, and the two discuss how dumbfounded they are by Jaxon's behavior. His mom recounts her assurances of a replacement toy and failure to discipline her son. His dad thinks she should have immediately taken away all of Jaxon's video game systems and then grounded him for a month, or even threatened to send him to military school. Both feel lost.

What happened here?

The parents worry Jaxon is becoming a "bad kid." They had really been trying to indulge him with new toys and more freedom with his time. Instead of being grateful, he has acted entitled, selfish, and even violent. They know he's been traumatized, but that was weeks ago, and the symptoms they originally saw—him being sullen and sleeping all the time—seemed to fade. They assumed that his anger was solely about his sister and the PlayStation, but although both twins were upset, only Jaxon resorted to violence.

Parents need to keep in mind that behavior like this can be a trauma symptom—one that isn't necessarily preceded by minor misbehavior. In fact, major misbehavior has more in common with being triggered (see Chapter 5) than the cries (or whines) for help inherent in some of the behavioral changes covered in the preceding chapters.

But why is this?

As discussed in Chapters 4 and 5, trauma reminders can trigger someone in a way that activates the fight–flight–freeze response by making the body think it is in danger. In a similar way, our anger—or any strong, overwhelming emotion—can activate the part of our brain that controls this instinct. Both Campbell and Jaxon felt anger about their sister's accident, but only Jaxon was unable to control it. Kids who are experiencing trauma symptoms are more prone to this type of reaction. The little voice in your head that, say, reminds you that your sister is just a little girl who had an accident and not a major threat isn't loud enough to overcome the pounding animal instinct activated by anger.

You can probably remember a time when someone cutting you off on the freeway had you on the verge of ramming their bumper—an overwhelming sense of anger seemed to temporarily overtake the usually logical, thinking part of your brain. In traumatized children, this dynamic arises with much greater frequency, especially when it comes to anger.

However, it is important to realize that the anger here doesn't necessarily stem from the traumatic event. Because they've been exposed to trauma, kids are simply more prone to outbursts from everyday stressors than their nontraumatized counterparts. To make matters worse, it's not just the trauma; it's their age, too. The prefrontal cortex of the brain, which is responsible for impulse control, isn't fully developed until people reach their mid-twenties.

Parents get caught up and don't know what to do in situations like this, as with Jaxon's parents' uncertainty over whether to appease their son or punish him. Unfortunately, neither tactic helps address major misbehavior in the long term. In fact, the wrong response may inadvertently reinforce the bad behavior. So, what are parents to do when their kids are acting out?

The solution is a four-part process: make sure everyone is safe, ground yourself, connect with your child and help the child calm down, and finally, set boundaries.

First: Get Safe

Before anything else, make sure that nobody gets hurt. For Jaxon's mom, this means separating him from both of his siblings.

For younger kids, like Jaxon, this can mean taking your misbehaving child to a safe space where you don't have to worry about anyone or anything getting hurt. Ideally, this will be a room without much stimulation and without objects that can be destroyed or used to cause injury. This not only gives your child the opportunity to calm down, but also grants you the opportunity to emotionally prepare yourself for the steps ahead. If you have a child who is frequently misbehaving in aggressive ways, consider setting aside one place in your home where the child can go and be safe even before regaining emotional control.

If you have a bigger kid who is actually at risk of seriously hurting someone else or themselves, don't be afraid to call for a spouse, trusted neighbor, or even a mobile crisis outreach team to come stand by your side. If Jaxon were sixteen instead of nine, his mom would have been smart to call for some backup. This will often be difficult. When I worked in an inpatient mental hospital, it was routine practice for every available doctor to show up when a patient was in acute crisis and acting out in a way that scared others. That show of support can require a major effort but is a powerful tool for calming the situation.

Second: Ground Yourself

Once you're confident that nobody is in serious danger, take a beat for yourself. The step after this is connecting with your angry child, and you need to be in the right head space to do this effectively.

Seeing your child threaten someone else with a balled-up fist or start wreaking havoc in the home is probably enough to make you feel scared and freeze up or want to run away—or even respond with anger of your own. These are natural and totally understandable responses. But they risk sending the wrong message, either that this behavior is acceptable, if you fail to address it, or to spark more of it by responding with over-the-top emotion. Your job in the moment is to lower the temperature, and you can't do this if you're not in the room, if you're mentally checked out, or if you're adding heat of your own to the situation.

So before anything, it is of critical importance to check in with yourself. You need to be calm and in control of yourself so that you help your child settle down. Sometimes this can simply mean taking a few deep breaths (remember: in through the nose and out through the mouth), splashing some water on your face, or using the classic DBT strategy of squeezing an ice cube. To read more about DBT, see the section on different therapeutic approaches in Chapter 11.

Also, many of the skills introduced in Chapter 5 (5-4-3-2-1, diaphragmatic breathing, progressive muscle relaxation) can also be used to help ground you, the parent. As stated above, even if you're not traumatized, your body can react to your child's violence in the same way the child's body reacts to his intense anger or to a trauma trigger. Strong, overwhelming emotions like anger and fear can kick off a cascade of physiological reactions that prime your stress response. Accordingly, you can use the same tools whether guiding your child through a trauma trigger or helping yourself calm down after that child has tried to beat up on a helpless sibling.

When explaining this dynamic to parents, I often tell them to think of themselves as like Luke Skywalker training with Yoda to become a Jedi Knight. At one point in his training, Luke must enter a cave where the dark side is strong. "What's in there?" he asks the wise Jedi Master. "Only what you take with you."

To be honest, I routinely see parents struggling to get this right. Parents are people too, and it is perfectly normal for them to feel overwhelmed or upset when seeing their child threaten violence. It takes practice to get it right. Often parents catch themselves in the middle of an anger outburst that can rival their own child's and must remind themselves to calm down and support their child—sometimes even using some of the relaxation training techniques that they had learned for the child's benefit.

Third: Connect and Calm

With that in mind, once everyone is safe, the next step is to connect with your child. Often this means making a basic statement of empathy. Something like "You seem very angry" or "Wow, you're upset" can be the right thing to say.

Tone here is important. It should sound like you're curious about their feelings and not just some all-knowing parental figure ready to pass down judgment. If you get this right, your child should soften a bit.

This simple connection opens the door to everything else. It shows that you are paying attention to your child and that you care. As a result, your child no longer feels alone with her emotions. Rather, she will begin to feel the strong foundation you provide as a parent.

Of course, this connection might not happen immediately. Anger is a powerful emotion, and a child's fast-beating heart and overworked limbic system may take a while to calm down. Sometimes children—especially young ones—can't get there on their own. I'll never forget the sweet four-year-old I saw for major misbehavior who, in one session, kept alternating between screams and sobs, fearfully yelling, "I don't know how to calm down!" Young children often don't know what to do with intense anger and may even get more distressed feeling these powerful feelings and the accompanying physiological response. This is where you come in. Again, some of the same skills used for responding to triggers in Chapter 5 can be used to help your child calm down during a period of intense anger. Think of diaphragmatic breathing, progressive muscle relaxation, 5-4-3-2-1, mindful walking, and the other tactics we have covered (see pages 87–95 for detailed descriptions of how to introduce and practice these skills with your child). As explained in Chapter 5, these skills can activate the parasympathetic response, helping kids calm down and regain control of their bodies and minds.

If you feel like you're not making progress, don't overdo it. Pushing too hard might further anger your child. Instead, give the child some space and let him know you're waiting—keep the door open and let him come to you. This isn't just about the right way to reach your child. There's no need to subject yourself to anger and verbal abuse from a child you love. Recognize your child's feelings, take a step back, and tell your child you're right there waiting for the child to calm down.

However, if you do have to take a step back, make sure to set boundaries about appropriate behavior. You can always help the child calm down more after the boundaries have been set.

Finally: Setting Boundaries

Once you've made a connection with your child—or at least taken the first steps toward connecting—it is important to reassert a hard line about what is and isn't appropriate behavior. Make a quick and short statement to show where the line is. For example, Jaxon's mom might say something like "I know you're mad, but in this house we keep our hands to ourselves."

It can be tempting to frame this line in terms of what your child shouldn't be doing: "Don't hurt people" or "Don't break things." Those statements are obviously true, but using negative terms like *don't, stop,* and *can't* sometimes has a way of inspiring pushback from children. It is a cliché for moody teenagers to growl, "Don't tell me what to do, Mom!" But things become clichés for a reason—because they happen all the time. You can sometimes circumvent a child's instinct for opposition by setting the boundary as a positive value rather than as antagonistic (see the box below).

Negative versus Positive Framing

Framing things in the positive does not come naturally to most people, and it can take some practice to make it habitual so that you use this language in the heat of a moment of major misbehavior. Consider these examples to get more comfortable with this framing device:

- "Don't punch holes in the wall" versus "Respect our home"
- "No hitting your brother" versus "Keep your hands to yourself"
- "Stop kicking the dog" versus "We're kind to animals in our family"
- "Quit starting fights at school" versus "Treat your classmates with respect"

However, if you're struggling in the moment to find the right positive framing, it is still *much* better to say no than to hesitate and let the behavior continue. It would have been perfectly fine for Jaxon's mom to have responded with "I know you're upset, but it is not okay to hit your sister." Your statement should validate your child's feelings, but not the misbehavior.

The important thing is that you're setting a boundary and standing by it.

You don't need to take too long setting this boundary or delve too deeply into what is happening. A single sentence will do. For example, if your son is ripping apart his sister's Barbie dolls, try "I know you're upset, but in this house we respect each other's property." Right now, your goal is to draw an immediate line around inappropriate behavior in a calm yet uncompromising way. It may seem like a small task, but the impact on a child can be immense.

But What about Time-Out and Other Punishments?

Parents may be tempted to let out their own feelings by yelling at their child or dispensing punishment. But this is the wrong step. You want to discipline your child, not punish them. When we discipline, we teach our children proper behavior. Just look at the word itself: The Latin root of discipline is *discipulus*, meaning "disciple" or "student." Punishment, on the other hand, stems from the Latin word *punir*, which means "to take vengeance." You should aspire to be a teacher for your child so that they act better in the future, not a vigilante seeking revenge for their bad behavior.

So how can you teach your child to be better? The first step is teaching her how to regain control after a blowup. In the last chapter, we talked about why selective attention and praise are so useful in addressing minor misbehavior. Parental attention is the strongest motivator of child behavior. However, this only works when a child is still in control. If your kid is back-talking or being sassy, her brain's protective layer of logical thinking is still working just fine.

But once the fight–flight–freeze instinct is in control, withholding your attention isn't going to help. If your child is exhibiting major acting out, as discussed earlier, the limbic system is running the show, and any attempt to instill proper behavior simply won't have a lasting effect. In this moment the child is not capable of internalizing lessons—and in fact pushing too hard might exacerbate the child's anger or undermine the connection you have just built. That's why it is so important for you to help your child calm down. Once they're back in control, they can learn the lesson you're going to impress upon them. Helping your child calm down also inherently teaches them the skills they can use to maintain self-control even in stressful situations.

This doesn't mean I'm suggesting you forgo consequences. There should be consequences for a room trashed or a wall with a hole punched in it. It does mean, however, that you should let go of any idea that you're going to successfully reprimand your child while the child is in a fight–flight–freeze state. Once your child has calmed down is the appropriate time to talk about consequences. As discussed in Chapter 7, consequences should be directly related to the offense perpetrated to maximize learning. For Jaxon, this might mean loss of privileges around his gaming system, not grounding him from social activities for a month or sending him to military school as his father was thinking of doing. Time-out is also a perfectly acceptable consequence—provided your child's trauma wasn't related to being confined in a space by himself. Time-out works best for toddlers and young children (six and under). For an effective time-out, your child should be in a room with minimal stimulation (or, if this is not possible, the corner of a room) for one minute for each year of age (for example, three minutes for a three-year-old). During the time-out, the child should not receive any attention—remember, attention is the biggest motivator of child behavior. If the child escapes, escort them back without talking until the time is up.

Responding to major misbehavior can be tough for some parents—unlike kids, adults have a more sturdy and developed cortex, but we're still vulnerable to emotion and anger. Just remember that you have a short-term goal (stop the major acting out) and a long-term goal (prevent it from happening in the future). To accomplish these goals, you need to interact with your child as he is and recognize how his brain is working—and not working. The steps we have covered might not come naturally for all parents, but they will help you curb major misbehavior.

You'll find a list of *dos* and *don'ts* for responding to major misbehavior near the end of this chapter. It's not a bad idea to refer to this list whenever you feel you've been at a loss for what to do when your child is acting out in a big way.

What Caused the Major Misbehavior?

In my experience as a therapist, instances of traumatized children engaging in major acting out are less frequent than other types of behavioral changes. When I do see kids threatening to hurt people or damage property, it isn't usually the result of trauma alone. Rather, trauma combined with some other problem has left them unable to control themselves when confronted with feelings of anger. These other problems can be as simple as not getting enough sleep or having enough to eat. Sometimes the problems are bigger, such as untreated health conditions or drug and alcohol abuse. These issues of personal well-being combine with trauma symptoms to make kids physically and mentally fragile, which loosens their grip on the fight–flight–freeze response and makes them more prone to explosive major misbehavior.

I once saw this dynamic play out in an unmistakable fashion with a six-year-old patient named Jayden. He and his mom had to leave their home due to domestic violence. As a result, they lacked permanent housing for weeks on end and had to share housing with other families. Jayden didn't have a bed to call his own. Meals were erratic.

Calm was hard to come by. When I first saw Jayden, his behaviors were entirely out of control. Normally kids act reserved when they initially meet a therapist. Jayden, on the other hand, was throwing books across the room and even tried to run out of my office. I ended up taking him to an empty safe room where we could calm down together. His behavior didn't change much as we began our regular sessions, until one day Jayden showed up with a smile on his face and an excited mood. After asking a few questions, I learned that Jayden's mom had finally been able to find them a new place to live—one where Jayden had his own bedroom and no noisy roommates. His major acting out disappeared the moment his basic needs were met. He still had other trauma symptoms, such as difficulty with concentration and impulsivity, but his destructive streak quickly ended.

Sometimes major misbehavior stems from problems with sleeping and eating. Often in teenagers I'll see newfound drug or alcohol abuse after a traumatic event that results in a child's sudden turn to violent or dangerous behavior. While other trauma symptoms usually have a direct connection to the original traumatizing event, major acting out is rarely caused by just one thing—it is a combination of several factors that leaves a child less able to control himself.

So if your child is engaging in major misbehavior, once you've responded by connecting, setting boundaries, and calming down, go through this mental checklist and see if anything pops out at you.

- **Drugs and alcohol:** Mind- and mood-altering substances leave kids less able to regulate their emotions. The slurred joy of a drunken stupor can quickly turn to rage. After all, there's a reason bars employ bouncers. Beyond the immediate effects, consumption of some drugs (including marijuana) can inhibit the long-term development of teenagers' growing brains—especially their prefrontal cortex, which is implicated in impulse control—and in turn makes them less able to control their emotions as they become adults. Finally, underage use of drugs and alcohol is illegal and might result in legal consequences that can inflict cascading harms on physical and mental health.

• **Sleep:** Insufficient sleep leaves us all vulnerable to irritability and little blowups. Combine that irritability with trauma symptoms, and you have a recipe for major misbehavior. Simply getting enough sleep can make a body more resilient to everyday stressors. Trauma hyperarousal symptoms, such as feeling jittery and overreacting to triggers, often make it difficult for kids to fall asleep. Consider helping your child with basic best practices for sleep hygiene, such as setting a regular bedtime routine, using the bed only for sleeping, avoiding caffeine in the afternoon, and turning off screens at least thirty minutes before bed. If noise or light is interfering with a good night's rest, consider getting your child blackout curtains, a white-noise machine, or earplugs. And if your child still has trouble sleeping, remind her that tossing and turning in bed can only make matters worse. Help her feel free to get up in the middle of the night and engage in a nonstimulating activity (reading a calm book, applying lavender-scented lotion) outside of bed before trying again to get some shut-eye.

• **Food:** Is your child having regular, healthy meals? Low blood sugar and insufficient nutrition can leave children feeling ragged and primed for a big outburst at a minor stressor. Don't worry too much about whether your kid is getting the fanciest organic foods. What matters is that he is eating something filling at regular intervals. Even a simple bowl of cereal and milk can do the trick.

• **Exercise:** A lack of healthy exercise can deny the body an easy source of natural mood boosters that help regulate anxiety and depression emotions. Getting up and moving around makes people more resilient to daily stresses and more able to control potential outbursts. Sometimes a daily walk can help get the body what it needs.

• **Connection:** Much of this book is already devoted to the parent–child relationship, but connection to same-age peers is also important for traumatized children. Because angry blowups might isolate a child from friends, it is important that you support your kid in repairing ruptures caused by anger and also in making new social connections. It may be necessary for you to find settings where your child can build these new connections. If so, build on your child's strengths. For example, if your nonathletic son is really into theater, choose acting classes or a community theater group rather than the sports team to help him find a new social circle. While making friends with same-age peers is something that is ultimately only in your child's control, you want to set him up for success.

Some of this advice may seem a bit simplistic. That's because it is—or at least it's simple. Often when you see the most extreme misbehaviors it is because something is going wrong at the most fundamental level. The brain can't control its base animal instincts if its basic needs aren't being met. And let me assure you, in my experience as a therapist I have never seen a child engaging in major acting out who wasn't also suffering from problems in one of these key essential areas.

Dos and Don'ts for Responding to Major Misbehavior

Here's a wrap-up of the advice given in this chapter as a handy reminder you can refer to when needed.

Do:

- Prioritize safety: Before anything else, everyone needs to be safe.
- Call for backup: Don't be afraid to reach out for help if you need it.
- Take a moment for yourself: Calm yourself before responding to the child's misbehavior.
- Connect before you correct: Connect with your child and help them ground themselves before you reassert a boundary or talk about discipline.

- Set boundaries: A close parent–child relationship doesn't mean you should forgo strong boundaries around major misbehavior. Physical aggression and destruction of property is never okay.

- Frame boundary-setting statements in positive language whenever possible.

Don't:

- Meet anger with anger: Scaring your traumatized child into good behavior will further damage your relationship.

- Go it alone: Responding to major misbehavior can be overwhelming to parents. If you can't call for backup immediately, be sure to debrief with a spouse, friend, or other supportive person.

- Neglect basic needs: People of all ages are vulnerable to angry outbursts when we are hungry, tired, lonely, or under the influence of mind-altering substances. Make sure that your basic needs and your child's are being met.

If your child is engaging in dangerous or destructive behavior, then professional therapy is likely recommended. But you as parents also have a critical role to play in confronting major misbehavior as it occurs, setting boundaries and keeping a watchful eye out for other underlying problems that could be leaving your child less capable of regulating their emotions. It is important to also remember the biophysical underpinnings of this type of misbehavior, which flows from dynamics similar to those discussed regarding triggers in Chapter 5. This is different from the motivating factors behind minor misbehavior, covered in Chapter 7, even if both are different types of misbehavior. Understanding how this works can be the key to your child's successful healing from trauma.

10

Responding to Self-Harm and Impulsive Behaviors

I once heard a parent describe raising a teenager as like being a member of NASA ground control on one of the early Apollo missions. "As our brave astronauts enter orbit into the dark side of the moon, we will temporarily lose contact with them here on Earth," he said, doing his best Walter Cronkite impression. "We can only hope and pray for their safety until they return."

As your kids grow up and begin to assert their own independence in middle school and high school, usual avenues of parent–child communication may start to fall silent. But for adolescents who have experienced something traumatic, it can seem like they're not only on the dark side of the moon, but blasted completely out of orbit, unmoored from the people and activities that used to keep them relatively stable. Instead they may begin engaging in impulsive and dangerous behavior.

This behavior may look like drug and alcohol abuse, self-harm, risky sexual habits, unsafe driving, shoplifting, running away, or skipping school. We call these *impulsive behaviors*. These types of troublesome practices overlap to some extent with major misbehavior—just picture an angry teen taking a swing at his father after Dad tried to reprimand him for coming home drunk. But there are key differences. Major misbehavior is an antagonistic, outward expression of the swelling frustration that can develop following trauma. When impulsive behavior occurs after an adverse event, it is often an attempt to silence or numb the internal stress brought about by trauma. Another difference: You can't miss major misbehavior—it's in your face and often aggressive. On the other hand, you may not realize your child is engaging in impulsive behavior until they get in a car crash or call you from the back of a police car after getting caught shoplifting. The teenager attacking his father was engaging in major misbehavior, but the drinking that preceded the altercation might have been impulsive. If his dad hadn't been waiting up for him, the drinking may have gone unnoticed and the physical altercation missed entirely.

Of course, teenagers can engage in these sorts of behaviors whether or not they've been traumatized. But there is a critical difference between typical teenage impulsivity and a response to trauma. In the former, kids are frequently motivated by social pressure, a pursuit of independence, and an earnest sense of fun and curiosity. In the latter, teens are often trying to find a distraction from the emotional pain or symptoms of trauma and an immediate relief from painful trauma-related thoughts and feelings.

Please also note that while the majority of this chapter focuses on older children and teenagers, younger children can also feel overwhelmed and experience a need to escape from painful trauma-related thoughts and feelings. The reason we often don't see the same type of impulsive behaviors in young children is lack of access (it's harder for them to get their hands on a bottle of alcohol, for example) and general fear of some of the impulsive behaviors. Running away or cutting seems a lot scarier to a six-year-old than a sixteen-year-old. Additionally, their same-age peers aren't engaging in this type of behavior, making it seem all the more strange and terrifying.

Typical Impulsive Behaviors

So what, specifically, does impulsive behavior look like following a trauma? In my practice, I routinely see three major categories of impulsive behavior among traumatized teens: drug and alcohol abuse, risky sexual habits, and self-harm.

Drugs and Alcohol

As noted above, drug and alcohol use can be common in middle and high school even when trauma isn't in the picture. Research shows that the vast majority of kids consume alcohol at some point prior to their eighteenth birthday, and just about half have tried drugs on at least one occasion. Think of beer at parties and sharing marijuana in the back of a car. If you find your child engaging in this kind of behavior, it can be tough to determine whether the child is expressing trauma symptoms or just displaying delinquent behavior. Again, one telltale difference is whether the behavior is social. Teens without trauma will typically consume drugs or alcohol in group settings, such as with friends or at gatherings where the combination of peer pressure, easy access, and genuine curiosity makes for a slippery slope. Traumatized teens may also consume drugs and alcohol in social settings, but a child who is regularly turning to drugs or alcohol in isolation (in addition to any social use) may be using it as self-medication to help deal with trauma symptoms. This looks more like smoking marijuana alone in the bathroom, stealing Mom's benzodiazepines from the medicine cabinet, or secretly experimenting with other intoxicants, such as huffing nitrous oxide from whipped-cream containers next to the refrigerator after everyone else has gone to sleep.

Risky Sexual Behavior

Risky sexual behavior is another classic example of impulsivity in traumatized teens. Sometimes the excitement and pleasure of sexual interactions serves as an effective distraction from trauma-related stress. Other times a child's self-esteem is so low that the child impulsively tries to trade sex for love and attention. However, it's important to keep in mind that there is a difference between risky behavior that poses a legitimate threat to your child's well-being and sexual behavior of which you simply do not approve.

For example, you may worry if you find a roll of condoms or a sex toy while cleaning up your daughter's bedroom, but this does not necessarily indicate she is engaging in a high-risk sexual behavior. In fact, it may be the opposite—she may be trying to safely explore a compelling biological imperative. So how do we define high-risk sexual behavior? Much of the research about high-risk sexual behavior in adolescents focuses on four key practices:

- Unprotected sex
- Sex with more than four different partners
- Participation in transactional sex
- Unassertiveness in refusal of sex acts

The common thread of these behaviors is that they put your child at serious risk of getting pregnant (or impregnating someone), contracting a disease, or even being exploited. Parents should also be aware that children who endured sex-related traumas can be at higher risk of engaging in dangerous sexual behavior. For example, I once had a client who changed schools after experiencing a sexual assault on campus. Despite things starting off well at her new school, she was eventually caught engaging in public sex several times with different partners on school grounds. Her behavior was more than normal teenage hormones and curiosity; it was a response to trauma. This type of pattern will be explained further under "Specific Trauma Type," later in the chapter.

Self-Harm

Nonsuicidal self-injury, or self-harm practiced without the intent to die, is another type of impulsive behavior we see in traumatized kids. I rarely see parents more distraught than when bringing in a child who is engaging in self-harm. They see cuts on arms, burn marks on legs, and they worry that their child is going to end up in the morgue. These concerns are normal. But in my experience as a psychologist, there is a complex list of reasons adolescents engage in self-harm, and many of these reasons have little to do with suicide.

While it can be difficult to understand the desire to hurt oneself, the physical pain inherent in self-harm also works to overwhelm and distract from the negative feelings associated with a trauma. Anyone who has ever hit the gym with extra gusto after a stressful day understands how overwhelming physical sensations can be an effective distraction. Consider a teenage girl who blames herself for missing a phone call from her closest friend, who then went on to commit suicide. She may stay up for hours at night ruminating about her failure to be there for her friend and is only able to distract herself from these painful thoughts and feelings through intense physical sensations, such as cutting her skin. Research shows that about one in four girls deliberately self-harms prior to her eighteenth birthday, and about one in eight boys does the same.

How Trauma Compromises Decision Making

These impulsive behaviors may all sound quite different: What does drinking have to do with cutting? However, the underlying cause stems from similar psychological conditions, and the way you approach them should be similar as well.

But first we must understand the pathway between trauma and impulsive behavior.

In Chapter 9, we reviewed how an underdeveloped prefrontal cortex can pair with the physiological mechanisms responsible for trauma triggers to result in a maelstrom of explosive misbehavior in traumatized children. Impulsive behaviors engage the same parts of the brain. The prefrontal cortex plays a major role in impulse control—whether we are talking about a child's impulse to strike a younger sister for ruining a gaming system or the sudden decision to shoplift a pair of shiny new earrings. But impulsive behaviors have an additional component: children's perception of their ability to cope. Many teens believe they simply cannot tolerate their painful, distressing trauma-related thoughts and feelings. In a strategy of avoidance, they may respond with impulsive behavior that distracts and overwhelms the emotional pain.

For example, I once had a teen patient who had impulsively run away from home without her phone or wallet. Police found her hours later, miles from her house, dehydrated and in a dangerous neighborhood. It turned out that a video of her being sexually abused—a potentially traumatic event in itself—had just been brought to her parents' attention. Her running away was a typical impulsive response to the shame and stress she experienced. Yes, it was a thoughtless teenage decision stemming from an underdeveloped prefrontal cortex. But she was also avoiding talking with her parents about something that felt shameful to her, attempting to escape after feeling triggered, and trying to avoid thinking about people and places that might create further stress for her. Running away allowed her to leave all of those worries behind, and the exhilaration of having a new experience and breaking the rules served as a powerful distraction.

In working with parents, I try to help them think about this kind of puzzling child behavior with one question: What is the function of the behavior? When it comes to distinguishing between normal teenage impulsivity and a trauma response, figure out why they're doing it: Is your child drinking because it's fun? Cutting herself because she saw a TikTok video about it and felt curious? Engaging in high-risk sex so he can brag about it to his friends? Keep in mind that social pressure can be a powerful motivator. If the risky behavior is merely social, then you'll still need to set some boundaries around it. If, on the other hand, your child is engaging in risky behaviors because they are stressed out and trying their best to cope, to avoid trauma-related thoughts and feelings, or to numb themselves, then they're probably exhibiting a trauma response that calls for your skillful support and therapy.

But how is a parent to know the function behind the behavior? Your teen is not likely to be forthright about his motivations for stealing your Ambien or drag racing, but you can use the principles discussed in Chapter 2 to help guide your thinking. Just like when we are looking at eating or sleeping habits to try to gauge whether our child has been traumatized, we want to compare his behavior to his baseline. If it was typical for your child to stay up long past bedtime playing video games before experiencing an adverse event, it's not so troublesome now to notice that his sleeping patterns are erratic. In the same way, it shouldn't be troublesome if your daredevil of a child is engaging in impulsive behavior. On the other hand, if your child tends to be more of a wallflower and suddenly starts sneaking out to drug-fueled parties, this is an indicator that trauma-related distress may be playing a role.

Other Risk Factors for Impulsivity

Of course, not every teen spends weekends chugging beers, racing cars, or engaging in other dangerous behaviors. In the same way, not every traumatized teen will engage in risky, impulsive behavior. You're more likely to see traumatized kids who share certain characteristics engage in these types of activities.

Age

Again, older teens have easier access to the people and products that can facilitate dangerous, impulsive behavior. A thirteen-year-old is less likely to impulsively participate in a drag race than a seventeen-year-old with a driver's license and access to a car. Alcohol, drugs, weapons, and high-risk sex are easier to come by as kids enter high school and cross the threshold into young adulthood. Having same-age peers—or even older ones—who engage in these types of behaviors (as is common in many teen social circles) also normalizes the behavior, making it less scary and threatening to do something that previously seemed scary.

Underlying Conditions

Traumatized teens with certain preexisting mental health conditions may have had a history of acting impulsively even before their exposure to a traumatic event. These conditions include borderline personality traits. Borderline personality disorder is a mental health condition characterized by instability in self-image that can manifest as trouble in relationships and difficulties managing stressful situations and emotions. People living with borderline personality traits may have a history of behaving impulsively in stressful situations, and adding trauma to the mix will exacerbate this tendency. Other underlying conditions, like attention-deficit/hyperactivity disorder, or ADHD, are also associated with impulsivity.

Specific Trauma Type

Sometimes the impulsive behavior has a relationship to the underlying trauma. While many traumatized children will try to avoid reminders of their trauma, others might feel inexplicably drawn toward their triggers. This can happen for a couple of different reasons. First is the human tendency to be drawn to the familiar. For nontraumatized kids, this might manifest as wanting only mac and cheese for dinner every night. Familiar foods can bring a sense of comfort and safety to your little one. For a traumatized teen, this might look like seeking out a dating relationship with someone who reminds them of an abuser. Remember in Chapter 1 when we talked about how trauma can shatter a child's view of herself, others, and the world? That is happening here: The world feels like a dangerous, scary place, so turning toward the familiar—even if it's abusive—can feel safe and predictable. Additionally, with sexual trauma in particular, teens may feel compromised self-worth, which can lead to unsafe sexual practices. This may track back to schemas (introduced in Chapter 1). For example, if a girl who was gang-raped at a party previously thought "good things happen to good people, bad things happen to bad people" and "girls who have sex with multiple partners the same night are gross," she might conclude she is a gross, bad person. I have treated many teen girls who feel worthless after sexual trauma and then engage in high-risk sexual behaviors like unassertiveness in refusing sex because they don't feel they are worthy of respect or believe the only way someone will show interest in them is if they are willing to engage in sex acts.

A Desire to Master the Trauma

Another reason teens might engage in impulsive behavior similar to their trauma type is a desire to master their trauma. For example, a kid traumatized by a physical assault from a school bully may impulsively start provoking other would-be bullies in an attempt to win a fight. A child who lost his home to a fire may suddenly feel drawn to matches and lighters. A teen who got into a serious car accident might speed down a highway one wet night in an attempt to "get it right." While this dynamic undoubtedly cuts down on avoidance symptoms, it may lead to unsafe behaviors and retraumatization.

Lack of Healthy Outlets

One reason adolescents engage in impulsive behavior is to distract themselves from emotional pain. Healthy outlets, such as playing a musical instrument, participating in sports, or having some other hobby, can serve the same functions without the risk. Teens who don't have these outlets are more likely to feel the need to engage in less healthy, more readily available distractions.

There's little parents can do about many of these risk factors. You can't change your kid's age or turn back the clock on trauma. However, there is one thing that you can control: providing your child with healthy outlets.

Never did I see this in such stark terms as when I was leading a therapy group for self-harming teen girls with trauma. The girls all came from different backgrounds, but they all had totally disengaged from any type of fun, esteem-building activity. Each one spent after-school hours either alone in her room or under the watchful eye of a caregiver. The girls had a lot of downtime and not a lot of opportunities to build on their strengths and foster a sense of confidence in themselves.

This situation wasn't necessarily the fault of their parents. Some of the girls had been pushed by their parents to get involved in time-filling, confidence-building activities, like karate lessons or church choir. However, it just didn't click. Pushback or even mere disinterest was enough to discourage the parents. That's an understandable response, but parents and teens alike need to recognize the link between positive activities and the ability to regulate emotions following a trauma. More information about how to do this will be provided later in this chapter. But for now, parents should keep in mind that this pushback may be another manifestation of trauma-related avoidance, as discussed in Chapter 8.

While avoidance symptoms might start out as evading people, places, and situations that actively remind the child of the adverse event, those symptoms can snowball into fears and avoidance of any stimuli if a child has been isolated enough. Think of a child who grew afraid of dogs after a vicious dog attack. At first, he was just afraid to walk around his neighborhood, the place where he was attacked. But after weeks of intense avoidance, he was afraid to be outside anywhere for fear a dog might show up and hurt him. Kids like this boy, or the girls in my self-harm group, weren't staying locked up in their rooms because they found it fun or compelling. They did it because it felt easier than getting out in the world, where they might be exposed to trauma triggers.

Responding to Impulsive Behaviors in the Traumatized Child

You now know why some traumatized teens turn to impulsive behaviors and what factors might make your traumatized teen more vulnerable to them. Let's take a look at a typical case of a traumatized teen acting impulsively and think about how his parents might respond:

Jordan is a senior in high school with fine grades and a great best friend. They had both earned basketball scholarships to a nearby university and were excited to play together. However, after the end of their senior-year basketball season, Jordan's friend was diagnosed with a late-stage cancer and passed away suddenly. Jordan was understandably shocked and devastated.

While Jordan's parents were glad he eventually started leaving his room and going out on weekends, they were puzzled about not seeing any of his friends around the house or hearing Jordan talk about them. Jordan's parents didn't worry too much because their son had always been so responsible and typically surrounded himself with ambitious peers who had impressive college plans of their own. But one Friday night the sound of a loud bang in the front yard scared them out of bed. They rushed outside to see Jordan's car smashed into the garage door. When they helped him out of the car, they noticed a strong scent of liquor on his breath, and it didn't take too long to realize their son had been drinking and driving. They were relieved that the only real harm seemed to be to the car and garage, but they were worried about what else could have happened.

What are parents to do in a situation like this?

Connection with Caregivers

First, the number-one goal for Jordan's parents should be to connect with their child. In the immediate aftermath of Jordan's drinking and driving, this initial connection should include making sure he doesn't have any injuries for which he would need medical care. Assuming he is physically safe at the moment, his parents can then shift to trying to understand where their son's drinking falls on the spectrum from occasional consumption to addiction.

Getting an understanding of Jordan's drinking behaviors may be difficult. Teens are already often reluctant to talk to their parents.

Shame around their impulsive behavior or fear of punishment could lead them to shut down even further. As you confront your child, do not approach him with threats or anger. Kids will pick up on that and clam up. Instead, think of yourself as Peter Falk's famous detective, Columbo. Even when he knew the answers, he would play ignorant, act curious about everything, and follow up with seemingly nonthreatening questions. With an attitude like that, it's no wonder California's elite criminals always talked. For Jordan's parents, this means not threatening to ground him or accuse him of anything. Instead, they should ask open-ended questions: What happened with you and the garage? Do you know anything about the liquor missing from the cabinets? This kind of questioning will help lead your child to drop their guard and open up. In contrast, launching accusations at children will just make them act defensively—even if (or especially if) the accusations are true.

Another idea you might try is sharing an example of a thoughtless, impulsive action you once took. This might look like "When I was sixteen, and your grandfather was out of town, I took his car without his permission to pick up some friends. Everything was going well until I hit a curb and popped a tire. I remember how embarrassed and terrified I felt. I was so worried he was going to kill me!" Parents might think that because their child broke the rules, they need to come down hard and fast, exuding disappointment and signaling a serious consequence is coming. Obviously your teen will be able to sense your judgment and anger, and this will not predispose her to openness. Acting like this will likely push your teenager into shutting down more. If you instead get a little vulnerable, she is more likely to meet you halfway, sharing her own thought process. You can still set a consequence for your child's behavior ("no more driving until you are sober and pay for the damages," for example), but your child is more likely to feel supported and be open with you if you can connect with her before you jump into discipline mode.

Sometimes even the most gentle, curious questioning and your own generous sharing can be met with an eye roll or a brush-off. If this happens to you, fear not. It could be part of your child's natural developmental process of seeking autonomy from caregivers, coupled with shame about the behaviors. In this case, it may be easier for your child to initially connect with someone more neutral—like a therapist—to ease some of the shame. Once your child has processed some of this with a therapist, the shame should start to lessen, and it may be easier to connect with you about what happened.

Before walking into a therapist's office, however, it's still important to connect with your child. If you sense he is unwilling to chat with you about the impulsive behaviors, it's better to connect via neutral, nonthreatening activities than to leave the teen alone. Aside from providing the child with connection, your physical proximity is helping to ensure your teen's safety until you can connect the teen with a therapist. A Friday night spent watching a horror movie with Mom is a wonderful alternative to spending the evening alone behind a locked door, where self-injury or cruising dating apps for hookups is more likely.

Not sure how to "be" around your child or what would constitute a "nonthreatening activity"? Flip back to pages 49–55 to review quality time, including a list of potential quality time activities. The fact teens are more independent than younger children doesn't mean they don't also need quality time with their caregivers. In addition to adding a barrier between your child and impulsive behaviors, one-on-one time will improve your relationship, helping your child feel more comfort in confiding in you.

Connection with a Therapist

While this book emphasizes that many kids who have been exposed to something potentially traumatic don't necessarily require therapy to heal, I typically do recommend therapy if your child is engaging in high-risk impulsive behaviors, if only because the consequences can be so dire. Getting a teenager to cooperate when scheduling a therapy session, however, can sometimes be difficult.

Not only do teens often have a gut instinct for independence, but teens who have been exposed to trauma often have some previous experience with therapists that might make them reluctant to sign up. For example, schools will routinely bring in a grief counselor for students after a potentially traumatic event. Sometimes this experience provides critical mental health support for kids in need and normalizes therapy in a helpful way. But sometimes the ordeal can lead teens to associate therapy with sitting in a sterile cafeteria surrounded by peers who couldn't care less—hardly a positive introduction to mental health services.

The trick here is to avoid power struggles when trying to connect your child with a therapist. Empower the teen as much as you can by offering choices: Individual or group setting? Man or woman or nonbinary therapist? Morning or after-school sessions? Don't feel like your child has to commit to the first therapist she sees. Trauma is often about loss of control, and the last thing your teen wants is to feel like she's losing even more control over the situation. See more about this in Chapter 11.

If your child is engaging in potentially dangerous and impulsive behavior, you need to be prepared to lend support when the child feels tempted to slide back into risky behavior. A therapist will help you and your child determine what this plan should look like. While you may know your child better than anyone, a therapist can provide an objective outside perspective, and also bring to the table the experience of someone who has handled situations like yours before. Parents may be reluctant to admit it, but even the strongest parent–child relationship is going to have some issues that teens are reluctant to discuss with Mom or Dad. Even Rory kept stuff from her mom in *Gilmore Girls*. And exposure to a trauma often exacerbates a teen's tendency to shut down (remember what we've covered about avoidance; see Chapter 8).

Safety Planning

A therapist can help with the development of a safety plan, which will allow you and your child to identify the situations and trauma triggers that lead to impulsive behavior, craft healthy, alternative coping responses, and think of supportive individuals who your child can turn to in moments of need. For example, Jordan's safety plan might involve recognizing how hearing his peers talk about college triggers worries of matriculating without his best friend. The plan will also involve teaching Jordan healthy coping skills such as diaphragmatic breathing (see the list on pages 87–95) and helping him reestablish once-strong relationships with his friends on the basketball team while also learning to rely on a guidance counselor at school, in addition to his parents at home.

This plan should also include adding healthy outlets to Jordan's life. With the loss of his constant companion and basketball season behind him, Jordan is adrift with nothing to fill the void in his life except for the painful memories of his traumatic loss. Alcohol instantly soothes this pain. However, Jordan can and should find other, productive ways to divert his attention and fill the gap in his day. This could involve joining an after-school sport league, volunteering at the local YMCA, or some other activity that aligns with his athletic talents.

By playing to his strengths, these positive distractions not only allow Jordan to avoid the immediate distress, but also build mastery and help him learn to cope over the long term. These diversions don't have to be anything particularly special or expensive; they just have to be a good for your child. Don't fret if your child is not an active, sporty kid like Jordan. Does your spirited son regularly sing in the shower? Maybe he'd be interested in voice lessons or joining a choir. Is your graceful daughter obsessed with the movie *Frozen*? Perhaps she'd enjoy ice-skating lessons. I once had a patient with awesome verbal comprehension skills who was able to manage her urges to cut herself by opening up the Duolingo language learning app every time she felt the compulsion to self-harm. By the end of our therapy together, she had not only mastered her posttraumatic stress symptoms but also reported that she was becoming conversational in Spanish. Still feeling stuck? This could be a good time to take your child on a trip to an art, hobby, or bookstore, walk the aisles, and see what piques her interest. Whether it's a sewing kit, a scrapbook, or a beginner's guide to yoga, go with your child's instinct.

In addition to finding activities that line up with your child's interests and strengths, you could find something that forges social ties with friends. If you can get your child to try some new activity that lines up with his interests, abilities, and social relationships, the intrinsic motivation for your child to keep it up should kick in. In other words, engaging in these healthy activities should feel good to your child and reinforce itself.

Finally, an effective safety plan will also likely involve a prevention aspect. If you're focused on decreasing self-harm and impulsive behavior, you need to become more aware of how your child engages in this behavior in the first place and create barriers between your child and the behavior. Jordan's parents, for example, might want to start locking up the liquor cabinet—or simply stop keeping alcohol in the house for the time being. For a kid who struggles with cutting, removing razors from the bathroom or putting a lock on the knife drawer can create an obstacle to impulsive action and give your child the time necessary to gain control over the fight–flight–freeze instinct that drives so much of harmful behavior. Kids will naturally bristle at these steps, viewing them as a kind of punishment. Parents may also be tempted to hand down harsh rules and reprimands in an attempt to punish their kids. However, as explained in Chapter 8, the goal here is not to punish your child. Rather, you are trying to teach the child how to control impulses and avoid serious risks to well-being. Whatever boundaries you place around your child, make sure they are the natural consequences of the impulsive behavior. Taking away Jordan's car after he crashes into the garage would be a natural consequence. On the other hand, something like forcing him to clean the gutters would be a poor fit and serve as mere punishment that does little to help him act responsibly with alcohol and driving.

Boundary Setting

Kids naturally bristle at boundaries, but if you engage with them in a fair, reasonable, and nonantagonistic manner, they're less likely to push back than children of parents who come down in a harsh, punitive, totalitarian way. For example, if Jordan's parents had demanded he be grounded for a month after discovering his drinking and car crash, we wouldn't be surprised to hear about him trying to sneak out of the house and get drunk, or even finding an alternate less-than-healthy distraction. On the other hand, if Jordan's mom let him know, in a nonantagonistic way, that she had to take away his car until they got his drinking under control to help keep him safe, Jordan would be more likely to understand this natural consequence and also be eager to address his impulsive behavior as a way to get his car back.

Setting boundaries in a nonantagonistic way may feel foreign to some. Most parents start out trying to set a boundary in a calm yet authoritative manner and are met by heated pushback from their kids. Being on the receiving end of that kind of attack is hard for many parents, but we want to meet their chaos with calm. As reviewed in Chapter 9, the most effective way to set boundaries is to leave our own anger out of it entirely. Then we want to reply with empathy, hold the line, and provide a short rationale for our boundary. This is what it might look like for Jordan's mom:

"Honey, I hear you're upset, and I know you want your car. I'm guessing it's a little embarrassing to have your mom drop you off at school. I need to take your keys, though, so that I can be sure you're safe while you're getting the drinking under control. Once you complete your program, we can talk about getting you the keys back."

This empathic response validates Jordan's frustration while staying firm in the decision to take his driving privileges away. There's also a very important benefit of setting boundaries this way: it preserves the parent–child relationship. Even if you are using all of the skills from prior chapters, if you blow up on your children after they do something impulsive, you're going to have a lot to repair. Responding with empathy and support while you hold the line won't do that kind of damage to your relationship and means you probably won't be having to set as many boundaries in the first place. A child who feels listened to and respected won't feel as many urges to push back against Mom and Dad's rules as one who feels punitively restricted.

Suicide Attempts

Sometimes children can engage in self-harm with the motivation to seriously injure themselves or end their lives. According to a 2019 study published by the CDC, 8.9 percent of children reported attempting suicide that year. These rates were significantly higher for children who identified as lesbian, gay, or bisexual, with nearly half of these children saying that they had seriously considered attempting suicide. Understanding the impact of trauma on suicide attempts is a bit more complicated. Rates of suicide attempts vary wildly based on the type of traumatic event, with physical abuse, sexual abuse, and neglect being associated with higher rates of attempts than other types of trauma. Additionally, rates of suicide attempts increase as abused children grow up and debilitating symptoms of posttraumatic stress remain untreated. Thinking back to Chapter 2, these are frequently the 10 percent of children who fall into the chronic symptoms category and require therapy and/or medication to facilitate healing.

Suicide attempts are frequently impulsive. Consider a teen girl who ran into an abuser on the way home from school overdosing on Tylenol because it was the first thing she saw when she ran to the bathroom sobbing. Other times, suicide attempts can be months in the making—a boy making plans to obtain a gun and shoot himself on the anniversary of his father's suicide, which is months away. Regardless of whether the attempt is an impulsive response to a trauma reminder or a long-term plan, a defining factor common to most suicide attempts is that the pain the child is feeling exceeds the capacity to cope. In other words, the trauma-related distress overwhelms all the child's resources, leaving the child desperate for relief. There are, of course, many other factors that play a role—including feelings of hopelessness, barriers to mental health care, and co-occurring mental health conditions—but this type of intense distress often accompanies these issues.

This is different from the impulsive self-harm teens engage in without the intent to die. If your child is talking about suicide or makes any type of reference to not wanting to live, this is something you should always take seriously. As with other forms of impulsive behavior, one of your first moves here should be to connect your child with professional help. A child who does not want to be alive anymore needs to be seen as quickly as possible. If you are unable to get your child in to see a therapist immediately, call a crisis outreach team, or if there are none available in your area, transport your child to a hospital for assessment and treatment. If you do not feel safe transporting your child and there are no crisis outreach teams in your area, do call your local emergency line and make it absolutely clear you need a mental health response. Until you are able to connect suicidal children with professional help, do not leave them alone. For more information on the services described here, flip to the Resources at the back of the book.

While other impulsive behaviors can be addressed simultaneously with trauma treatment, a child having suicidal thoughts and a plan to end his own life is a contraindication for many trauma treatments. Before we think about treating the trauma, the child has to be stable. The previous chapters have explained that many behavioral changes that take place following a trauma can be at least partially adaptive because they temporarily decrease the extent of the distress your child is feeling. As covered in Chapter 8, avoidance is so powerful because when children avoid what makes them feel anxious, their in-the-moment anxiety plummets. At the same time, their overall distress, and their perception about how well they can cope with distress, grows and grows. Treatment focuses on confronting the feared triggers, so that they are not so fearful of them and overall distress falls.

This would not apply to children who are actively suicidal. We want them to have all of their defenses, regardless of how unhealthy these defenses may be, because it is better than the alternative. For this reason, trauma treatment should be put on the back burner, at least until we can be confident these children are safe.

Bringing It All Together

Nearly all teens engage in risky behavior. They're driven by an instinct to seek independence and a desire for social connection with their peers. Meanwhile, a still-forming prefrontal cortex means that the logical part of the brain isn't at full capacity to help temper questionable decision making. Add trauma to the mix, with the accompanying struggle to tolerate distress and regulate emotions, and you are in for a wild ride.

As the parent of an older child or adolescent who has suffered a potentially traumatic event, it is your job to determine (along with your child's therapist and/or care team) whether involvement with drugs or alcohol, self-harm, or risky sex falls into the category of dumb but expected teen behavior or is a more serious response to trauma. Either way, you'll need to set some boundaries to keep your child safe. If you approach this in a nonpunitive, reasonable manner, you can keep your child close, rather than inserting more distance between you. Keep in mind that having the crucial benefits of a strong parent–child connection and enlisting a therapist to help with safety planning will go a long way in curbing these behaviors.

Responding to risky impulsive behavior is a difficult task given the average teenager's recalcitrance. But nobody said that being a parent was easy. Like one of those Apollo mission control scientists, it is your job to keep your astronaut safe, even if she is not always talking to you.

PART IV

Parenting Plus

11

Seeking Professional Help

As I've said several times in this book, most children impacted by adverse events will go on to heal naturally, without any professional intervention. If, however, your child seems to be struggling with the posttraumatic stress symptoms listed in Chapter 2 or the behavioral changes noted in Chapters 5–10 and these symptoms interfere with your child's everyday life, it's time to seek professional help.

When to Seek Professional Help

To review, here are the symptoms you should be on the lookout for:

- Hyperarousal symptoms, including jumpiness, difficulty with concentration, irritability, changes in appetite or sleep habits

- Avoidance symptoms, including trying to stay away from people, places, and things that remind them of the event, not being able to remember the event

- Intrusive reexperiencing symptoms, including nightmares, flashbacks, and distressing memories of the event

- Dissociation symptoms, like your child not having the feeling of being in his body

- Negative thoughts, like "the world is not a safe place" or "this was all my fault"

- Negative feelings, including fear, horror, anger, shame, or guilt

- Any other behavior changes that seem "out of the norm" for your child, including those covered in this book (major misbehavior, self-harm)

Don't panic if you notice your child experiencing any of these symptoms, even if they linger. The presence of these symptoms does not mean your child is destined to experience a chronic mental health condition. In fact, children of all ages can experience a low level of these symptoms at different points in life, all while achieving academic success, maintaining friendships, and being a functional part of their family system.

Still feeling confused about when should you get a professional involved?

The primary indicator that you should take action is whether or not these symptoms seem to be interfering with your child's day-to-day life, especially in the context of school, home life, or friendships, or in taking care of basic needs. Consider the following examples:

- Rosie, age seven, was traumatized after she was present while her father had a heart attack. She had a host of symptoms immediately following the heart attack, like difficulty sleeping, jumpiness, and nightmares, but those have since resolved. She has also had a hard time getting to school. While Rosie once loved school, she now cries throughout the morning routine and begs to stay home. At the latest parent–teacher conference, Rosie's teachers say she seems sad, worried, and distracted, remarking that she has been especially tearful in the months following her father's heart attack.

- Art, age fifteen, was traumatized after a school shooting. His mother was relieved that he never seemed fearful about returning to school but is concerned that her once social boy quit the basketball team and now spends his weekends alone in his room.

• Savannah, eighteen, was traumatized by a major car crash. Her father understood when she didn't want to drive in the following weeks, but six months after the crash he's getting tired of driving her to school and to outings. When he tried to encourage her to drive herself to an outing, with him in the passenger seat for support, she became instantly tearful and jittery, and he worried about her ability to drive safely given how jumpy she was with every lane change.

The common factor in each of these cases is that ongoing trauma symptoms are interfering with everyday life. For Rosie, it's her struggle to separate from her parents and her feelings of sadness and worry that are intruding on her time at school. With Art, his avoidance symptoms may have influenced his decision to quit the team, distance himself from his friends, and keep him isolated. With Savannah, her jitters are getting in the way of her desire to drive and her ability to drive confidently, a milestone she had excitedly achieved two years prior. Their parents of all three would be wise to seek professional help.

But where should they start? Most parents looking to explore therapeutic treatment options first consult Dr. Google. Surfing through website after website can feel confusing. It may seem like there is an entirely new language to decode in the quest to find an appropriate provider. Consult the glossary in the box on pages 186–187 for terms you're likely to come across when trying to make decisions about what therapy might be right for your child.

What Types of Therapy Are Effective for Traumatized Children and Teenagers?

Whether you're buying a new car seat for your toddler or trying to help your teenager pick a college, you know better than to simply go with the first option that comes your way. You do your research—look at ratings by outside groups, weigh the costs, and read consumer satisfaction reports. So should it be different with therapists? We should aim

A Glossary of Terms Related to Therapy Options

Clinical trial: A research study using human subjects. For different therapy approaches, clinical trials help determine if the therapies studied are effective and how they perform compared to other therapy approaches.

Cognitive therapies: Cognitive elements of therapy focus on the relationship between thoughts, feelings, and behaviors and demonstrate how unhelpful or inaccurate thinking can lead to painful feelings and unhelpful behaviors. Cognitive therapies generally focus on how changing thoughts can positively impact feelings and behaviors. In trauma treatment, this might include distorted thoughts like "I'll never be normal again" or "the world is a very dangerous place."

Efficacious: How well a treatment performs in ideal situations, like a clinical trial. This is different from how effective a treatment is in the real world, where therapy appointments might be interrupted or all components of a treatment might not be delivered exactly as intended.

Evidence-based practice: Therapies based on scientific evidence, like the results of clinical trials.

Exposure therapy: Therapies for trauma and anxiety that focus on approaching or turning toward what makes the client feel anxious, as opposed to relying on avoidance to decrease short-term distress. Typically done in a gradual manner, exposure can help decrease avoidance symptoms and long-term distress, often leaving clients feeling empowered to reclaim parts of their lives lost to posttraumatic stress.

Family therapy: Therapy that includes the members of a family. The goal is typically to improve communication and decrease conflict between family members, which may increase after an adverse event.

Gold standard: Therapeutic approaches or modalities (defined below) that are considered the best-performing treatments out there, according to research.

Group therapy: Therapy provided to several people at the same time, in the same place. The individuals in the group often have no prior acquaintance but may share the same types of problems for which they are seeking treatment (for example, trauma symptoms).

Individual therapy: Therapy provided by a therapist for one patient. Anyone else who joins a session (such as a parent) is there for the patient's benefit.

Manualized treatment: Therapy interventions that are performed according to specific, strict guidelines for administration, written by the developers of the therapy approach. Advocates for manualized treatment tout how this approach maximizes the likelihood of the therapy being performed consistently, regardless of who the therapist is.

Modality: The type of therapy. This can refer to the therapy itself (for example, TF-CBT, DBT) or to how it is implemented in a specific setting (for example, individual therapy, group therapy, family therapy).

Psychoeducation: A component of many different types of therapy. It specifically refers to teaching, typically about the mental condition being treated. In many trauma treatments, psychoeducation consists of teaching patients and their families about trauma, PTSD, the role avoidance can play in PTSD, and what posttraumatic stress symptoms look like.

Psychological assessment and evaluations: A series of psychological tests designed to help a psychologist better understand a patient's diagnosis or answer other questions about psychological functioning. Can be used on its own or in conjunction with therapy.

to be savvy consumers when getting therapy for our children the same way we would for any other service our child needs.

Part of being a savvy consumer is knowing what to look for. Some studies have shown that simply having a trained professional to talk to, without an agenda, can decrease symptoms of general mental distress. At the same time, the research is abundantly clear that some therapy approaches are more effective than others, especially when it comes to the treatment of child trauma. But with countless different types of therapy out there, where do you even begin?

Trauma-Focused Cognitive-Behavioral Therapy

Clinical research and my anecdotal experience are clear: Trauma-focused cognitive-behavioral therapy (TF-CBT) is the gold standard when it comes to the treatment of trauma in children. I recall remarking to a fellow therapist that it was "like magic" seeing almost every child who received the treatment experience a significant decrease in posttraumatic stress symptoms.

While there are individual differences between TF-CBT therapists, because it is a manualized treatment, the way the therapy is delivered will look similar and have common elements, regardless of practitioner.

If your child is seeing a therapist for TF-CBT, the first half of the treatment will focus on skill building. This includes components like psychoeducation about trauma, which will teach your child about prevalence rates of different adverse events and common ways children respond to trauma, helping to normalize their experience. Children will also learn relaxation training skills that can be used to help tolerate both trauma-related distress and everyday stressors. I once had a traumatized high schooler report back to me—long after the conclusion of therapy—that he used relaxation training skills learned in our TF-CBT therapy to successfully calm himself down before his college entrance exam.

In addition to psychoeducation and relaxation training skills, children receiving TF-CBT will learn skills around expressing and responding to thoughts and feelings that will aid them both in processing their trauma and in everyday life. In most cases, a supportive caregiver will be attending some of these sessions with the child; the child will teach the parent the skills he just learned, improving parent–child communication and reinforcing skill acquisition.

After the skill-building portion of treatment, the child and therapist collaborate on a trauma narrative that serves as a type of exposure and ultimately opens the door for processing any lingering thoughts that could be getting a child stuck in their healing (for example, "This was all my fault"). At the pinnacle of treatment, the child will share this narrative with the supportive caregiver who has been attending therapy with them. The narrative not only serves as exposure but also enhances the parent–child relationship so that the child feels better able to turn to the parent if they experience any trauma-related distress after the conclusion of therapy. The treatment frequently ends with work on enhancing safety, which can be an important part of future trauma prevention.

One Size Does Not Fit All

There are, of course, times when TF-CBT is not the best for a child or family. Perhaps, in the aftermath of an adverse event, a family is in too much chaos to attend the type of regular, consistent therapy necessary for a treatment like TF-CBT. For example, if a family lost their home to a natural disaster and is without a stable living situation, attending weekly therapy appointments might not be possible. Or perhaps you have an older adolescent, itching to establish himself, who might find the heavy parent involvement of TF-CBT a turnoff. Maybe your child has picked up an unsafe self-harm habit you'd like to address before addressing the trauma. Whatever the case is, it's important to keep in mind that TF-CBT might not always be the best fit for your child.

Here are some other evidence-based alternatives worth looking into:

For families needing more flexibility than TF-CBT provides, **Attachment, Self-Regulation, and Competency (ARC)** may be a better fit. ARC is a treatment program that obviously focuses on the three primary areas of attachment, self-regulation, and competency. Therapists identify "building blocks" or targets for the therapy within these domains. This process is intended to build toward integrating a traumatic experience in a healthy way that reduces problematic symptoms. If your home life is currently in chaos and consistent weekly therapy seems untenable, ARC might an ideal fit.

Cognitive processing therapy (CPT) is considered a gold-standard treatment for PTSD in adults but can also be effective in treating younger patients. CPT includes psychoeducation about trauma and focuses mainly on addressing those thoughts that can keep people from natural recovery. The therapy will identify these thoughts or "stuck points" and teach patients how to systematically challenge and replace them with more accurate, helpful thoughts. I recommend CPT for those older adolescents who are yearning for independence, and especially those who seem plagued by distressing thoughts like "I'll never trust anyone again" or "the world is a completely dangerous place."

For children and adolescents whose trauma symptoms are mainly manifesting through dangerous impulsive behaviors like self-harm or high-risk sexual behaviors, I often advise **dialectical behavior therapy (DBT)** before or in place of TF-CBT. DBT is a skills-based therapy that teaches mindfulness, distress tolerance, emotion regulation, and how to be effective in relationships, many of the domains that impulsive children and adolescents struggle with. It was originally developed for the treatment of borderline personality disorder, which overlaps with posttraumatic stress symptoms including impulsivity. This means it can uniquely target those risky, impetuous behaviors covered in Chapter 10. If you feel your child's impulsivity is putting her at risk of serious harm, I would advise starting with DBT. If, after the completion of DBT, your child is still experiencing posttraumatic stress symptoms that interfere with everyday life, TF-CBT or another trauma treatment can be started.

Mentalization-based treatment with children (MBT-C) would be my treatment of choice for parents struggling to form a secure attachment relationship with their child. If reading Chapter 3 of this book felt overwhelming to you, MBT-C is a great place to start. This short-term therapy treats parents and children and will help you and your child make sense of your own minds and the minds around you. In doing so, MBT-C promotes a closer parent–child relationship, leaving you and your child better able to make use of the skills in this book.

If your younger child (age two to seven) is struggling with minor and major misbehavior more than other trauma symptoms and this behavior is getting in the way of a close parent–child relationship, **parent–child interaction therapy (PCIT)** might be a better fit for your family. Parents learn effective relationship building and discipline skills. This process begins with teaching sessions between parents and the therapist. Then, using a one-way mirror and a "bug in the ear" communication device, the therapist coaches the caregiver in the specific skills learned in prior sessions as they interact in play with the child. This therapy will help curb behaviors covered in Chapters 7 and 9, from tantrums and back talk to destruction of property and physical aggression.

Whenever I see a child whose symptoms fall mainly into the avoidance realm, I often consider whether **prolonged exposure (PE)** for children or adolescents might be the best fit. If I ever see a child who is still experiencing avoidance symptoms after a course of TF-CBT, I always recommend PE as the next approach. Exposure is at the heart of this treatment that is comprised of imaginal exposure, which takes place in the therapy office and has the child recount the traumatic experience, and *in vivo* exposure, which has a parent accompany the child on exposures to feared people, places, and situations in the child's everyday life. Older adolescents may complete these exposures without parents.

If the adverse event bringing your child to therapy is related to grief and loss, **trauma and grief component therapy for adolescents (TGCT-A)** might be the best fit for your child. TF-CBT does have an adaptation for grief and loss, but not every TF-CBT therapist is trained in this. TGCT-A teaches many of the same skills as TF-CBT but addresses specific components of grief in a way that TF-CBT (without the added grief component) would not.

How to Find the Right Therapist

You're now familiar with many of the evidence-based treatments used to address trauma symptoms, but how do you choose a practitioner? I have three recommendations:

- Ask your child's pediatrician: Given the high prevalence rates of adverse experiences in children, your child's pediatrician is likely all too familiar with the best trauma-trained therapists in your area.

- Ask your child's school counselor: In large schools, the school counselors make referrals to outside therapists on a daily basis. This is another place to get trusted referrals.

- Consult the directory for the specific type of therapy you want: Many of the therapies covered above have training or credentialing processes and keep a directory with a running list of providers who are trained or credentialed in those modalities. See the Resources at the back of the book for links to some of these lists.

After you have identified a few therapists that seem like a good fit for your child, give them a call. You might consider asking about the following:

- Experience working with children your child's age
- Experience working with trauma and/or the specific type of adverse event your child has experienced
- Which modality is used
- Cost of sessions and whether insurance is accepted
- Hours of availability, including whether the therapist offers after-school appointments
- How the therapist thinks about parent involvement in therapy

Ideally, you will be able to select a therapist who meets your and your child's needs. If you've found multiple therapists and can't decide who to go with, don't sweat the decision too much. Since most trauma-focused therapies are manualized, your child's experience might not differ significantly based on who you choose.

Talking to Your Child about Therapy

I encourage parents of young children to frame their child's first visit to me as an appointment with a "talking doctor" who will help them talk about thoughts and feelings. I also encourage parents to give their children space to ask any questions they may have, such as "Can you come with me?" and "How long will it be?" to help ease appointment-related anxiety. Most therapists will be happy to hop on a quick call with you to give you more information about what the first appointment will look like so you can answer your child's questions.

For older children and adolescents, it might be helpful to start by saying that sometimes after experiencing a scary or stressful event, it can be helpful to visit with a therapist. Also give older children the chance to ask questions and space to express any mixed feelings or reservations they might have about therapy. Also give your children a chance to express any preferences they might have for therapy. If your older children are ambivalent about therapy, try consulting them about whether they would prefer a male or female therapist, what time they would like to have the sessions, and if they would prefer individual or group therapy (almost all of the modalities above can be offered on an individual or group basis). If giving choices doesn't work, encourage your child to try it out for one meeting. Sometimes a therapist can help resolve ambivalence about therapy if the child gets through the door.

Seeking Your Own Help

Being a parent is hard work. Parenting with love and patience can feel overwhelming, regardless of how your child's trauma symptoms manifest. Entering your own therapy can go a long way in alleviating some of the parenting stress. For many parents, therapy is one of the only times each week when the focus is on them and their needs.

If you notice any of the following symptoms, this could indicate you would benefit from your own therapy:

- Feeling preoccupied with thoughts of your child's trauma and how it can impact them

- Feeling exhausted, overwhelmed, or resentful of your child's minor or major misbehavior

- Feeling paralyzed with fear when your child acts in dangerous, impulsive ways

- Feeling annoyed or resentful about increased emotionality, behavioral regression, or avoidance symptoms your child is displaying

- Any of the posttraumatic stress symptoms identified in Chapter 2 that are interfering with your day-to-day life

Fear not if you feel like you don't "click" with the first therapist you speak to. As with your children, it's okay to call a few therapists before booking your initial appointment to make sure you select someone you feel good about. I would assert that perceived fit between therapist and client is even more important for adults. While therapy with traumatized kids is often about specialized skill building, parents in this situation typically just need some support. This means it is important to find a therapist who makes you feel comfortable and at ease, so don't feel like you must commit to the first therapist you call.

I almost always get some pushback when I recommend therapy to parents. They typically argue that they don't have the time, or that they don't need it, or that it simply feels selfish to focus on themselves with a suffering child at home. Nothing can be further from the truth. Therapy for a parent can very much be part of a child's healing process. Parents are the foundation of healing from trauma. If parents aren't emotionally strong, then this foundation risks crumbling. Therapy is what helps parents be there for their children—even if it means being somewhere else for an hour a week.

It's like the airlines' warnings during their safety announcements: If you ever hit a rough patch, put on your own oxygen masks first and then turn to help your kids.

Consider the example of Mia, an eight-year-old girl who had just survived an awful house fire.

Mia's second-grade teachers always used to comment on how precocious and funny she was. After she was in the fire, however, Mia started acting much more reserved and shut down. The school therapist began to see Mia, but progress was slow. It seemed like she wasn't getting the support she needed at home. The therapist eventually realized that Mia's caregiver, her grandfather Ralph, was a Gulf War veteran who had his own lingering traumas related to surviving the crash of a helicopter that burst into flames upon impact. This trauma made it hard for him to engage in her healing process. Every time Mia tried to talk with him about loud noises and lingering pain from the crash, he would simply try to change the topic or even get upset and leave the room. Mia's therapist eventually called Ralph in for a one-on-one meeting and recommended he find his own psychologist. Ralph was reluctant at first, but after seeing a therapist at the local VA hospital Ralph began to address his own avoidance symptoms. Now able to talk with her grandfather about her scary experience, Mia is back to her usual self at school. And Grandpa Ralph is starting to plan a fun vacation for the two of them—after all, he hadn't been on an airplane in thirty years.

Even if you don't have a trauma history like Ralph, hearing your child recount painful experiences can be overwhelming. In seeking your own help, you are doing something important for your child. You're making sure that you can be there for them and able to talk about the often scary or upsetting experiences that can be hard for parents to hear.

There is another major benefit from parents going to therapy: You're showing your child that it's okay to ask for and receive help. Sometimes parents think they have to seem invulnerable or perfectly stoic when their kids are watching—no crying, no getting angry, no appearing weak. But this idea of the perfect parent can actually be quite damaging to a child! You are your children's model for adulthood, and they will internalize your actions and behaviors as normal. So please, show your kids that it is normal to seek out help when you need it, ask for a hug when you're sad, and acknowledge your feelings in healthy ways.

But What about the Stigma?

Public normalization of psychological health services has come a long way over the past few decades. Whether it's veterans receiving help for posttraumatic stress, broader coverage by insurance, or millennials joking about their psychologists on Twitter, something that may have been viewed in a negative light is now widely accepted. However, stigma still exists in some places. This can be stigma from your community or your extended family, or internalized stigma from yourself for pursuing therapy.

Consciously or unconsciously, people might have a negative view of seeking services for themselves or their child. They might worry that it shows they're weak, that it means they've been bad parents, that they're wasting their time. Parents might be embarrassed to be recognized by someone they know in the waiting room.

Do any of these concerns resonate with you when you think about seeking therapy services for yourself and your child?

If so, don't fret. Worries like this are normal in our culture. Unfortunately, these sorts of negative thoughts can and do lead to a lot of people suffering in silence rather than getting the help they need. Anytime you hear your inner voice stigmatizing you, I encourage you to reframe some of those automatic thoughts.

Instead of "I'm weak for needing therapy," try on "I'm strong for doing what it takes to take care of myself and my family."

Instead of "I'm a failure as a parent because my child needs therapy," think "I'm being an attentive parent for responding so quickly to my child's needs."

It is your job as a parent to take care of your child. If you're able to march through this swamp of stigma to help your child, that just shows you're willing to do what it takes to get the job done.

Putting It All Together

If you take away one overarching lesson from this book, it should be that the best way to manage emotional distress is by connecting with other people to whom we feel securely attached. For your child, this most often means connecting to the primary caregiver(s).

Sometimes, though, a child's distress can be so intense that the average caregiver couldn't possibly know how to deal with the symptoms—say, major misbehavior or self-harm. Or maybe just dealing with all the usual burdens of parenting can make a child's trauma seem that much more overwhelming.

In these cases, it is important for you to show your child that even if you personally don't know how or are unable to immediately make things better, you do know the proper steps to address the underlying issue. You want it to be obvious that you care, you're trying to help, and you have a sense of whom you can contact—such as a therapist—to make things better.

The worst-case scenario would be a kid who is desperately acting out inner pain, begging for relief, yet emotionally isolated from caregivers. Make it clear to your kid that you hear them and that you are an authority and expert on what it takes to heal—and sometimes that means therapy.

12

Looking Ahead

When you decided to read this book, you were probably worried about your child. Maybe you were even concerned that exposure to a potentially traumatic event meant your kid would be scarred for life. By now you should know that's not true. You know that nearly all children have the capacity to heal. You also know that it may take some work. At this point, you may already be seeing encouraging changes in your child's behavior—tantrums have lost their steam, the bedtime routine has returned to normal, and parent–teacher conferences are all about your child's bright future instead of disruptive classroom behaviors. At the same time, some kids may need even more support from parents and professionals, and recovery can come slowly.

Whether your child is recovering naturally, exhibiting mild symptoms, or has been struggling with painful posttraumatic stress symptoms for an extended period of time, a traumatized child can go on to lead a healthy, productive life with help from a strong parent–child relationship, use of the skills in this book, and support from a professional if needed.

This recovery may seem incredible if your child is having a very hard time following an adverse event, but it is important to keep in mind that symptoms can always reemerge later in life. In fact, symptom resurgence is a normal part of the healing process, and I wish this fact were better known.

All too often I see stories in the media about people overcoming incredible adversity and going on to amazing achievements—a woman who runs competitively despite having seizures during races or a war photographer who continues to work after losing his legs in a terrorist attack. Stories like these can make us feel like even children who have the symptoms of PTSD just need to get "over the hump" of trauma and then they'll be able to thrive and live the rest of their lives unencumbered. Some people will even take away the message that enduring trauma will somehow build character.

Unfortunately, this isn't necessarily true. While there can be growth through adversity, enduring trauma and recovering from it doesn't ensure superhuman emotional fortitude or even preclude a return of symptoms. Expectations for posttraumatic flourishing may set up many of our kids to experience shame if and when some of their old posttraumatic stress symptoms pop up again. **But just as your kids relied on you to help them respond to the initial trauma, you can be the key to assisting them whenever symptoms return. And this time, you'll both be ready.**

There are many reasons that children may see a resurgence of symptoms, but some of the most common causes include: big life adjustments and changes (such as moving to a new city and starting at a new school), experiencing novel or infrequent triggers (the anniversary date of a trauma, for example), not taking care of basic needs (including sleep and nutrition), and chronic stressors (such as a toxic friend group).

I once had a five-year-old patient who had been separated from his parents during a long-term hospital stay. He recovered from the resulting trauma, only to struggle more than the average kindergartner after he started school that fall. Spending full days away from his mother terrified him and reminded him of their painful and scary separation, and his mom received a worried message from his teacher that he was spending most school days crying in a corner by himself.

When the fourteen-year-old girl I saw started dating for the first time after recovering from sexual abuse, she suddenly found herself triggered every time her boyfriend tried to hold her hand. For her, being triggered meant freezing and shutting down. He would ask her why her hand was always cold and clammy and why she seemed distant and checked out every time he tried to get close to her. Ultimately, he broke up with her, explaining that he didn't think she liked him very much. She was distraught and confused by her body's responses to mere handholding and didn't understand how the abuse she had healed from five years prior could still be impacting her.

Also consider the case of Shaiann, an eighteen-year-old college freshman who was traumatized five years earlier when her brother was killed by a drunk driver. Shaiann was extremely distressed by the loss of her brother and struggled with a host of posttraumatic stress symptoms, including difficulty sleeping, angry outbursts, and ruminating on the awful things she wanted to happen to the driver of the car. Her parents immediately connected her to a grief and loss support group, as well as individual therapy to treat her posttraumatic stress. Shaiann responded well to these interventions: She started sleeping better and noticed she was thinking less about the driver and more about how to honor her brother's memory. She even became a mentor at the treatment center where she attended support groups for kids who have lost family members. After she graduated from high school, her parents were worried about her going away to college, but Shaiann seemed to make the transition quite easily. That is, until Shaiann learned via a Google alert that the drunk driver who had killed her brother would soon be granted parole. Shaiann didn't have much to say on the phone when her parents called, and they thought she might just need some space. However, a few days later they received a worried call from Shaiann's roommate, who said she had been acting in a concerning manner—just that day, after spending time reading something on her laptop, Shaiann screamed an obscenity and threw her laptop against the wall before running out of the room without another word. Her parents guess that Shaiann's distress is related to the upcoming parole but are hesitant to reach out to her and inquire about this, for fear they might trigger her.

What can these children's parents do to help them from afar?

Forecast Returning Symptoms

Part of your child's healing from trauma—or any mental health condition—means recognizing that they may be vulnerable to symptom resurgence at some point in the future. The worst part is our kids can often be caught off guard by this relapse and feel frustration or even shame about experiencing painful symptoms they thought they had overcome. If you can clue them in ahead of time that hitting these bumps in the road is a normal, natural part of the recovery process, you can not only cut down on the shame but also prepare them to cope. Here's what you can do:

• Make it clear that it's normal to see some symptoms pop back up, especially when kids are going through changes in life, and that it's not a reflection of how well they did in recovering from their trauma. Studies have shown that over half of those who had been treated for PTSD later reported subthreshold symptoms—meaning some posttraumatic stress symptoms but not enough for the full PTSD diagnosis. If your children went to therapy as part of the healing process, a natural time to bring this up could be at the conclusion of therapy. Let them know they did a great job in therapy and that sometimes when life gets really stressful or a new trauma reminder pops up it's normal for some of the symptoms to return. Also let them know that if and when that happens they can always come to you for support or return to therapy for some booster sessions.

• If your child recovered without therapy, you might share a similar message when you notice the triggers have decreased and the other behavioral changes have begun to subside. For a new driver who was traumatized in a car crash, a parent might say something like "You've been doing so great driving to school every day. I know sometimes after people are in crashes like yours the fear can pop back up again. This could happen if you're under a lot of stress, or when it starts to snow again, like it was the day of your crash. If that happens to you, let me know. We could do some more drives together." This type of sentiment would be appropriate for the five-year-old described above, the college freshman, and everyone in between.

Be on the Lookout for Vulnerable Times

In addition to forecasting that symptoms may return after your child heals initially, you can be on the lookout for times he may be most vulnerable to a resurgence. Here's what to do:

• *Keep an eye out for trauma reminders:* You can anticipate moments when you might typically see symptoms flare again. Shaiann's parents might be looking for a possible resurgence of symptoms after they hear the news about the driver's release from prison. Other times symptoms might flare are on anniversary dates related to the trauma or upon hearing about a similar trauma befalling someone close. Symptoms can also return on birthdays of victims and during holiday celebrations and significant life events when a missing presence can be particularly palpable. If your child had a special Christmas tradition of playing football with his cousin who unexpectedly passed away last year, you might pay extra attention to your child's mood when December hits.

• *Think about non-trauma-related risk factors for relapse:* High-stress environments, abusing substances, and not taking care of basic needs all put your child at increased risk for resurgence of posttraumatic stress symptoms. Studying all through the night for tests, going off to summer camp, or matriculating at college are a few examples. While these events may not cause a symptom resurgence on their own, they make your child more vulnerable when a trauma trigger pops up.

- *Recognize early warning signs:* These may look different for different kids. With younger children, we are more likely to see behaviors like increased clinginess, physical complaints like stomachaches and headaches, increased tearfulness and behavioral regression, and minor misbehavior. For older kids, avoidance and withdrawal, substance abuse, self-harm, other impulsive behaviors, and sleep impairment may be more common. For most kids experiencing a resurgence of symptoms, their new symptoms may have a good deal of overlap with their original symptoms, though this is not always the case.

Model Seeking Emotional Support

Because avoidance is a hallmark of posttraumatic stress, it can be especially easy for symptoms to sneak up on children and disconnect them from their support system before they ever knew what hit them. Sprinkle some shame on top of this avoidance, and your child will be doubly isolated. I've frequently heard patients endorse thoughts like "I should be over this by now," which keeps them from sharing their pain with even their most trusted confidants.

Having a model for when and how to seek emotional support can go a long way toward showing children it's okay to reveal vulnerability to others. You can be this model. We all undoubtedly have stress in our lives, and our kids are pretty good at picking up on this no matter how we may try to hide it. Show your child it's okay to ask for help by seeking out your own support when you're stressed. Whether you have a close friend you go to for advice or you're in therapy of your own, don't hesitate to mention it to your child.

You don't have to make a big deal of it, but next time you notice you're feeling stressed, saying something along the lines of "I could really use a coffee date with Aunt Barb right now; that always makes me feel better" or "My therapist said the most interesting thing today . . . " can demonstrate to your child that it's good to seek support as needed.

Talk About, Normalize,
and Validate Feelings

For a young child fearful of starting at a new school, this means talking about how new events can be scary—and maybe you were once afraid of starting a new job or moving to a new state. If you sense your younger child is fearful about a transition like this, make some space for the child to express those feelings. Something as simple as "How are you feeling about starting school?" could be sufficient, or fall back on some of the ideas (such as roses, buds, and thorns) from Chapter 6. Creating a routine to facilitate sharing of everyday thoughts and feelings around the dinner table can go a long way.

If your child shares feeling nervous about starting at a new school, normalize and validate that feeling, as explained in Chapter 6. This could sound like "I bet any kid starting a new school feels a little nervous" or "I remember feeling terrified the night before I started high school."

A young teenager dealing with a reemergence of old trauma symptoms connected to her history of sexual abuse while dating new, age-appropriate partners could use a reminder that jumping into a new relationship is scary for everyone and it is important to listen to our bodies and communicate with partners. At the same time, a fourteen-year-old may not feel comfortable discussing the intricacies of her romantic relationship with Mom or Dad. Consider encouraging the conversation by saying something like "How are things going with [boyfriend]?" If your teen then hints that things are not going well, continue with something like "I bet a lot of girls who've had scary experiences like yours have feelings about starting a new relationship. If that's the case for you, I'm here to talk, or I could call Dr. [therapist] if you like."

A young woman like Shaiann might be afraid to talk to her parents about her feelings stemming from the drunk driver's parole out of concern that it would upset them. Her parents were also simultaneously worried that bringing it up to Shaiann would trigger her. But

what we know about this situation is that Shaiann may have been triggered either way: It's not the talking about it that's most triggering; it's
the fact that this man is being released from prison in the first place.
Shaiann will eventually learn about the parole. Better that she hear
it from her parents than from a Google alert. After her parents share
what they've learned about the parole, they might ask how she feels
about it. No matter what she's feeling—angry, sad, confused, numb,
or any other way—her parents should try to understand, then normalize and validate these feelings ("It makes sense that you feel furious.
There are a lot of people in our family who feel the same way" or "Our
family has been through the wringer, and it makes sense you'd feel
numb and tapped out").

In most cases, a resurgence of symptoms is less distressing than
the original trauma symptoms your child experienced. This means
your child probably will not need another full course of therapy or for
you to review all the skills covered in this book in depth. What these
symptoms do call for, however, is skillful support.

If you recognize a symptom resurgence in your child, you might
say something like "That's three nights this week you've had nightmares—how stressful for you. Do you think it could be time for a
booster session with Dr. [therapist]?" or "Would you like to practice
some belly breathing tonight before bed?"

Bringing It All Together

Parenting a traumatized child can seem overwhelming and terrifying.
But at present, and in your child's future, you have everything you
need to help your child.

At the heart of this help is the parent–child relationship. As
stated at the beginning of the book, the best way any of us can cope
with emotional pain inherent in trauma is by connecting with the
people we feel most securely attached to. For your child, that means

you. Using the skills covered in Chapter 3—amping up quality time, mentalizing, praise, active listening, and enjoyment—and cutting down on commands, judgment, and sarcasm will propel your relationship with your child forward.

A strong parent–child relationship also means your child knows she can turn to you not just for emotional support, but also for the know-how to cope with strange and painful new trauma-related feelings. This is where the skills in Chapters 5–11 come in. You know what to do:

- If your child is being triggered, use the grounding and relaxation exercises covered in Chapter 5.

- If your child is increasingly emotional or is experiencing a behavioral regression, reinforce them for talking about their feelings and load them up with validation, physical touch, and extra attention as covered in Chapter 6.

- If your child is exhibiting an increase in minor misbehavior, use selective attention and praise skills outlined in Chapter 7.

- If your child is withdrawing from friends and family due to anxiety about posttraumatic stress, think about how exposure can help manage the impacts of avoidance, as reviewed in Chapter 8.

- If your child is misbehaving in a major way, aim to connect with your child before you correct her and then set a firm boundary in a positive way, while also making sure her basic needs are being met as covered in Chapter 9.

- If your child is engaging in risky, impulsive behaviors like substance abuse, unsafe sex, or self-harm, take a look at the skills in Chapter 10, including identifying healthy outlets and safety planning.

- And if you don't know where to start, or worry your child may be struggling, consider the types of professional help outlined in Chapter 11 to get your child connected with extra support.

Armed with a secure attachment, the skills taught in this book, belief in your child's own inherent ability to heal, and, if necessary, professional support, you can set and keep your child on the road from traumatization to empowerment.

Resources

Helpful Apps

Breathe
- Available only on the Apple Watch, this app uses animation to help guide people of all ages through deep, calming breaths.

Breathe, Think, Do with Sesame Street
- Aimed at children ages two through five, this app is focused on emotional development and relaxation training skills.

Breath Ball Breathing Exercise
- Designed for ages four and up, this app uses visual imagery to help guide different breathing exercises, including those that can help when a child is triggered or struggling to sleep.

Calm
- For children four and up, this app includes sleep stories and meditation guides.

Moshi Kids: Sleep and Meditation
- This app is used by children of all ages and launches new meditations and guided imagery each Wednesday. These can be used to help children calm down after a trigger or wind down for bedtime.

Super Stretch Yoga
- A yoga app designed for children of all ages, to be used conjointly with parents or without, Super Stretch Yoga uses storytelling and animation to teach kids yoga. This can be used as part of quality time or as a relaxation and grounding skill.

Wellemental: Kids Mindfulness
- Designed for ages four and up, this app provides guidance in yoga, sleep, and guided meditations. Can be used together with a parent, or alone as grounding skill, anger management, and distraction.

Helpful Books

To read with your child:

Burton, L., Bernardo, S. S., & Fletcher, C. (2014). *The rhino who swallowed a storm.* Burbank, CA: Reading Rainbow.

Holmes, M. M., & Pillo, C. I. (2000). *A terrible thing happened.* Washington, DC: Magination Press.

Karst, P. (2000). *The invisible string.* Camarillo, CA: DeVorss Publications.

Penn, A. (1993). *The kissing hand.* Indianapolis, IN: Tanglewood Press.

To read on your own:

Allen, J. G. (2008). *Coping with trauma: Hope through understanding.* Washington, DC: American Psychiatric Publishing.

Hagelquist, J. O., & Rasmussen, H. (2020). *Mentalization in the family: A guide for professionals and parents.* London: Routledge.

Harris, N. B. (2018). *The deepest well: Healing the long-term effects of childhood adversity.* Boston: Houghton Mifflin Harcourt.

Hayes, S. C. (2005). *Get out of your mind and into your life: The new acceptance and commitment therapy.* Oakland, CA: New Harbinger Publications.

Hoffman, K., Cooper, G., & Powell, B. (2017). *Raising a secure child: How circle of security parenting can help you nurture your child's attachment, emotional resilience, and freedom to explore.* New York: Guilford Press.

Lansbury, J. (2013). *No bad kids: Toddler discipline without shame.* Malibu, CA: JLML Press.

Siegel, D. J., & Bryson, T. P. (2011). *The whole-brain child: 12 revolutionary strategies to nurture your child's developing mind.* New York: Penguin Random House.

Siegel, D. J., & Bryson, T. P. (2016). *No-drama discipline: The whole-brain way to calm the chaos and nurture your child's developing mind.* New York: Bantam.

van der Kolk, B. A. (2015). *The body keeps the score: Brain, mind, and body in the healing of trauma.* New York: Penguin Books.

Helpful Contacts

Crisis Text Line: Text HELLO to 741-741 (U.S.)
Lifeline Crisis Support: Call 13 11 14 (Australia)
National Suicide Prevention Lifeline: Call 800-273-8255 (U.S.)
National Teen Dating Abuse Helpline: Call 1-866-331-9474 (U.S.)
NHS Childline for Suicidal Thoughts: Call 0800 1111 (U.K.)
RAINN National Sexual Assault Hotline: Call 1-800-656-4673 (U.S.)
YoungMinds Textline: Text YM to 85258 (U.K.)

Helpful Websites

Websites for certified and rostered therapists in evidence-based treatments for trauma:

Find a rostered CPT therapist
- *https://cptforptsd.com/cpt-provider-roster*

Find a certified PCIT therapist
- *www.pcit.org/find-a-provider1.html*

Find a certified PE therapist
- *www.med.upenn.edu/ctsa/find_pe_therapist.html*

Find a certified TF-CBT therapist
- *https://tfcbt.org/therapists*

Websites with parenting resources:

American Academy of Child and Adolescent Psychiatry
- *www.aacap.org/AACAP/Families_and_Youth/Resource_Centers/Disaster_Resource_Center/Resources_for_Parents_Disaster.aspx*

Black Emotional and Mental Health Collective list of mobile crisis services in the United States
- *www.beam.community/mobilecrisis*

Child Trauma Academy
- *www.childtrauma.org/trauma-ptsd*

Child Welfare Information Gateway
- *www.childwelfare.gov/topics/responding/trauma/caregivers*

Institute on Violence, Abuse, and Trauma
- *www.ivatcenters.org*

Lifeline (Australia)
- *www.lifeline.org.au*

National Center for PTSD
- *www.ptsd.va.gov*

National Center on Substance Abuse and Child Welfare
- *https://ncsacw.samhsa.gov/resources/trauma/trauma-resource-center-websites. aspx*

The National Child Traumatic Stress Network
- *www.nctsn.org*

Nemours Children's Health
- *www.kidshealth.org/en/kids*

Nemours Teen's Health
- *www.kidshealth.org/en/teens*

PCIT International
- *www.pcit.org/for-parents.html*

Zero to Three
- *www.zerotothree.org*

Index

About the Author

Melissa Goldberg Mintz, PsyD, is a clinical psychologist in private practice in Houston, Texas, and Clinical Assistant Professor at Baylor College of Medicine. Dr. Goldberg Mintz is passionate about providing evidence-based care to children, adolescents, and adults who have experienced trauma.